The Color of
GRAY

(Living and Dying with Alzheimer's)
(Types of Abuse and Sexual Relations)

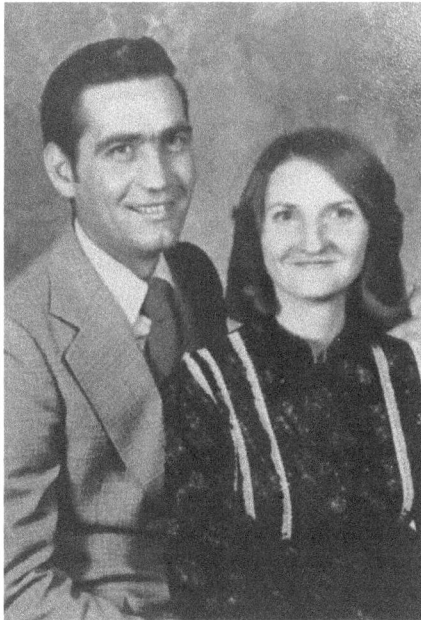

2nd Edition

The Color of
GRAY

(Living and Dying with Alzheimer's)
(Types of Abuse and Sexual Relations)

Polly Lynch Spainhour

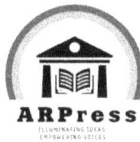

ARPress
ILLUMINATING IDEAS
EMPOWERING VOICES

ARPress
45 Dan Road Suite 5
Canton MA 02021
Hotline: 1(888) 821-0229
Fax: 1(508) 545-7580

Ordering Information:
Quantity sales. Special discounts are available on quantity purchases by corporations, associations, and others. For details, contact the publisher at the address above.

Printed in the United States of America.

ISBN-13:   Paperback   979-8-89389-032-7
           eBook   979-8-89389-033-4

Library of Congress Control Number: 2024910124

Table of Contents

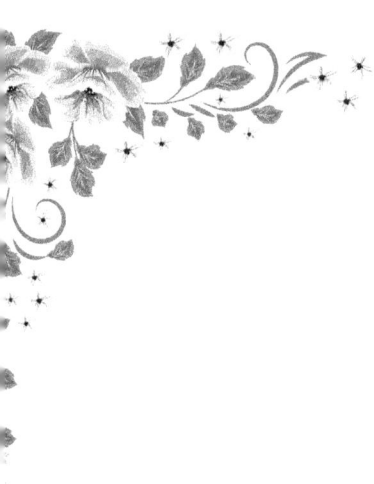

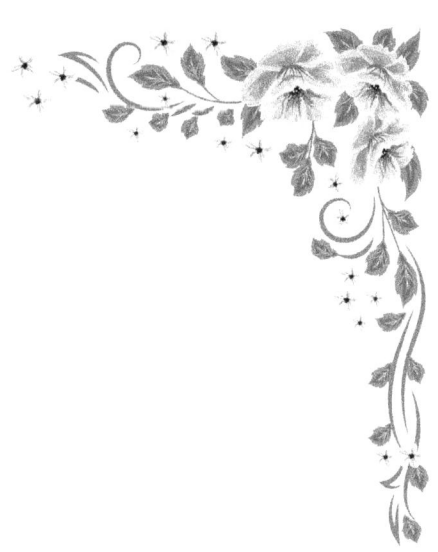

For all victims of Alzheimer's
And their caregivers

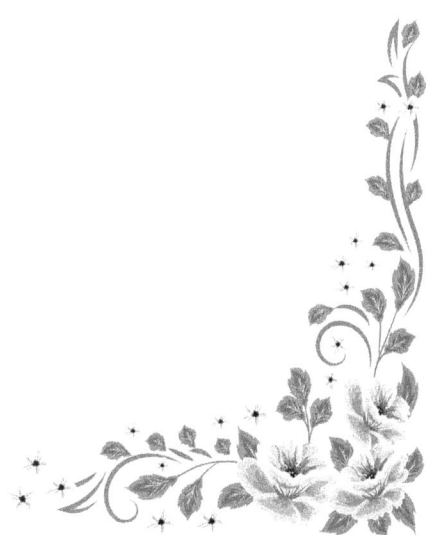

PROLOGUE

I began keeping a journal of things my husband said and did, when he was forty seven. At that time little was known about Alzheimer's. People who had not come face to face with this monster, chose to be in denial. They also hoped it would go away. I didn't understand things that were happening, and felt if I told anyone what was happening, I would not be believed. I did, and they didn't.

There were many things that happened, are still in my memory, but I chose not to share them. Some names have been changed. My prayer is that something said in this book will touch and help someone else. After the first publication, I was humbled with tears, and thanks for sharing.

I especially wish to thank Donna Tilley for her support and friendship throughout the duration. I have received lots of encouragement from many people in different ways. You know who you are and I thank you.

Glenda Walters, a dear friend and fellow author with whom we have shared dreams, thoughts, and tears; Kaye McCormick, who has helped keep me sane, and who can soothe a weary soul; Laverne Gordon, who was a fellow graduate from high school and a retired librarian with years of expertise. She has been a helpful source of knowledge; Ralph and Gail Key, who could write a book of observations during this trying time; Anna Nichols, Lizzie Saunders, and Dewey Sturdivant, with the Pilot Mountain Charles Stone Memorial Library, have been willing to answer questions, or to refer me to the appropriate contact person.

I, also, wish to express thanks to my family for their love and support throughout the years. Even though they didn't understand some of the choices that I made, they were still there for me.

Last, but definitely not least; thanks are immensely given for the continued, effortless endeavors of Ms. Zoe Parker (Author Advisor), and Ms. Angela Paige (Fulfillment Officer), and CEO Miquel Hernandez's comments.

All the scriptures used are from the authorized King James version.

Writing poetry was an outlet for me, if just for a moment. I have included several poems in this book. These will give you an insight as to how I was dealing with a situation at that particular time. Then, again, you may wonder, where in the world was she?

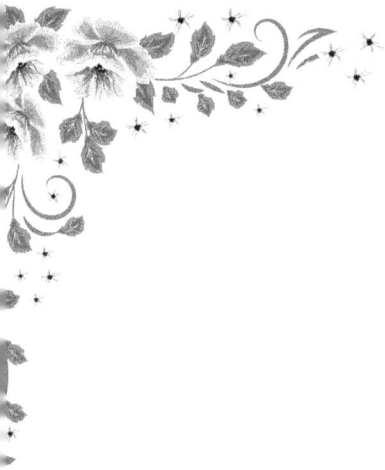

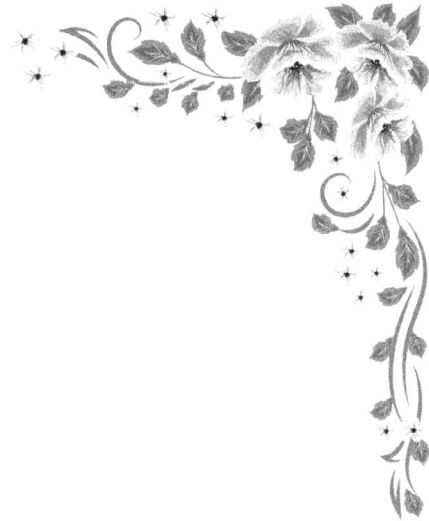

I have been asked "What are the signs of Alzheimer's," by many people over the years. Before Ken was actually diagnosed, I had read several books trying to figure out on my own what was happening. Now, we have the computer where we can have instant access to, as the old saying is "whatever ails you." I would suggest going on Internet and typing in "symptoms of Alzheimer's." This will give you the early signs and answer a lot of your questions. Ken was diagnosed as being in the final stages in 1998, and lived until 2007. Other individuals may not do so. Each situation is different.

For those of you who do not have access to a computer, the following guideline came from the Aricept Caregivers Guide to Alzheimer's.

THE STAGES OF ALZHEIMER'S

BEGINNING - MILD STAGE
Has memory loss
Forgets names of common objects
Asks the same questions. Repeats the same things, over and over
Gets lost easily
Loses interest in things he/she once enjoyed
Loses things more often than normal
Isn't acting like the person you know

MODERATE - SEVERE STAGE
Has trouble remembering recent events
Has trouble with simple tasks, like dressing or washing dishes
Forgets to shave or shower
Argues more often
Believes things are real, even when they are not
Wanders, often at night
Seems worried/depressed

SEVERE - FINAL STAGE
Cannot use or understand words
Cannot recognize self or family members
Cannot care for self

Since the first publication of this book, questions have been asked. The information that I am sharing is from reading for many years, people sharing, and my own experience.

" REMEMBER I AM NOT A DOCTOR"

Often, there is *"an elephant in the room"* in a marriage. This is evident when either, or both, are no longer interested in each other's sexual needs. Many *"baby boomers"* were prohibited from asking about their biological *"private parts."* It was therefore challenging to express emotions or questions. The younger generation has more awareness of a wide range of issues, frequently at an early age.

I decided to bring this up in the conservation right now for a purpose. Put your thinking cap on. There will undoubtedly be some people who say, "I thought this was about Alzheimer's." It is hoped that the couple's sexual relationship has been fulfilling. Maybe not. It's possible that the person is unable to communicate with their feelings. Most of the time, the spouse who is providing care has a lot of unanswered questions. That's the least of our worries, people will say.

As the individual becomes more, and more less communicable, this leaves the caregiver needing that hug, support, or bond. For some people, this may not be a problem, but to others, yes. As a caregiver (spouse) you have enough to focus on. Some medical specialist presents the individual, and spouse with helpful information. Others, do not. There are books available, but all people aren't aware which book to buy. There is a well written book entitled **Naked at our Age.** The author is *Joan Price.* There may be sections you choose to not read. Skip over. Before you laugh, this is needful for your physical and emotional health. Ask/..! Talk to your doctor. Most insurance companies will cover regular therapy. Ask.

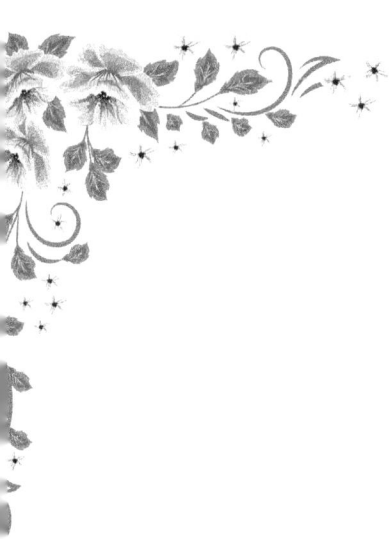

BEGINNING – MILD STAGE

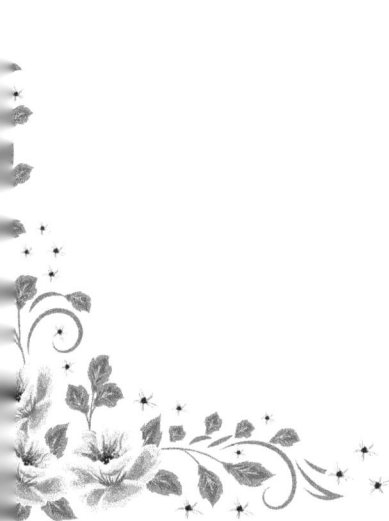

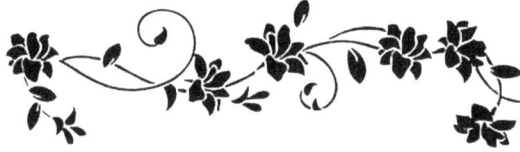

SOMETHING'S AMISS

Where are you?
Where have you gone?
Why have you left me here all alone?
Night after night you leave me this way.
It leaves me so empty that I don't know what to say.
What did I do to be treated like this?
When we first met it was such wonderful bliss.
Everything could be solved with a kiss.
In my heart I can tell something's amiss.
What could be more important than us being together?
Is love like living through stormy weather?

03/1995

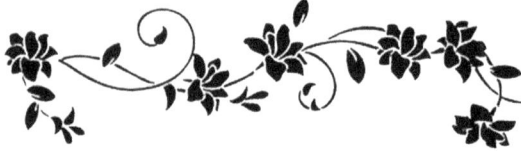

MY HEART IS LONELY

My heart is lonely without you.
I'm reaching out for you and you're no longer there.
You have slipped away again into your own little world.
Where have you gone?
What do you see?
What do you feel?
Do you want everything to be quiet and still?
What's in your mind?
What are you thinking?
You look straight ahead without even blinking.
Do you have pain anywhere,
and do you really care?
Are there things you can't face in the real world?
Are your thoughts in such a turmoil
that from true life you have recoiled?
You have left me out in the cold for so long.
Sometimes it's so hard to hang on
to what we once had,
and for me, that's rather sad.

04/25/95

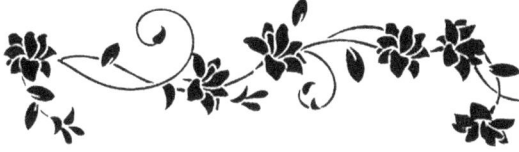

THE ELUSIVE BUTTERFLY

The butterfly emerges from its' chrysalis
and tries out new found wings.
Each butterfly is so unique;
it reminds me of a rainbow
when the colors are at their peak.
Like the gold at the end of the rainbow,
when you try to catch one—it's so elusive.
One minute it's there, and then it's gone,
leaving you wondering—what's going on?
Have you ever watched a child chase after a butterfly?
The air is filled with laughter as the little hands reach out
seemingly for the unattainable—but she still tries.

05/15/95

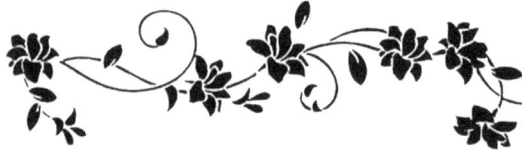

BUILDING CASTLES IN THE SAND

A child builds a castle in the sand
using nothing but his own little hands.
Maybe a bucket or two—even a shovel will do.
A little pat here, a little pat there;
so involved in his work and showing his derriere.
He works so diligently and innocently,
his concentration so sweet and mild.
He digs a moat around his castle
to keep out all that will harm.
When the waves wash it all away,
he's ready to rebuild another day.

05/22/95

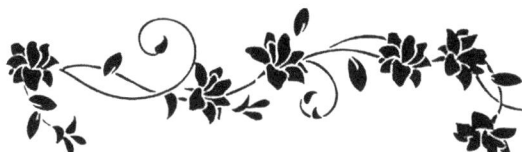

AFTER THE STORM

Lightning flashes across the sky
with jagged edges going from side to side
burning a path wherever it travels.
You look for somewhere to hide
trying to quiet the fear of your heart.
Your body is shaking as if hit by a dart.
Lightening travels back and forth
as it lights up the night.
For just a second the heavens come alive
with a maddening sight.
You hear the thunder rumbling in the distance
shaking the earth with little resistance.
A heart can be broken by harsh words
spoken in anger, just as the lightening
breaks open the firmament with its tremendous power.
A heart can be mended, but it will never be the same.
The sky will again be beautiful with the moon and stars,
but it will never be as it was…
before the storm.

06/08/95

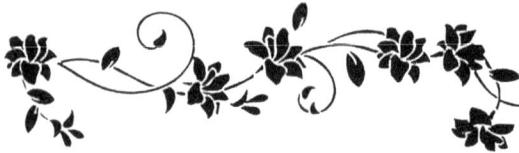

LEARNING ABOUT LIFE

My thoughts travel back to my childhood days,
and of my life that has changed in so many ways.
I wonder in my mind what might have been,
if I could live my life all over again.
Would I have the same friends?
Would I play the same games?
So many reflections are there for me to see;
how some people can hear while others are deaf;
how some people can see the leaves on the trees,
while others can only hear the rustle of the leaves;
how to plant seed and watch the crops as they grow,
and watching the water as over the rocks it flows;
catching lightning bugs with two small hands,
and watching them glow when put in a can.
Listening to the night sounds as I lay in bed,
when I should've been sleeping with dreams in my head.

07/28/95

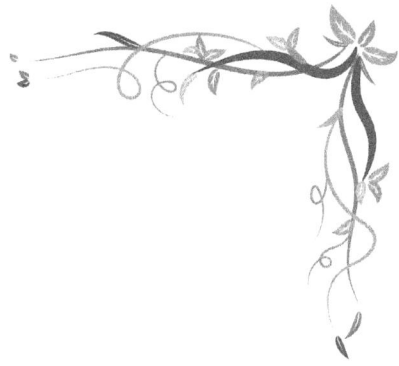

08/26/95

Ken stood quietly watching the neighbor's new white kitten, as she frolicked amongst the leaves with the nine year old calico cat. There was a look of bewilderment upon Ken's face as he asked, "When did Gail get the calico cat?" When I heard this, chills ran up and down my spine. Why did he not recognize the calico which he had known for so long? The feelings that I had kept rejecting now refused to be ignored. I finally had to admit something terrible was wrong with Ken. Thus, began our long and painful journey of living with this yet, undiagnosed monster, called Alzheimer's.

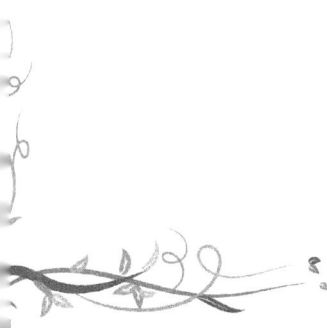

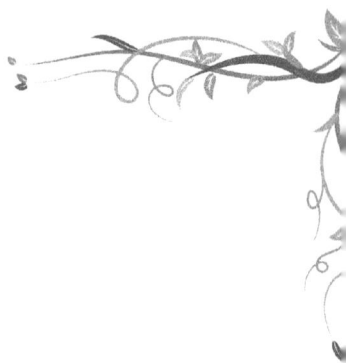

08/29/95

Saturday, Ken bought a box of potatoes, and left them in a chair on the carport. Monday was such a beautiful day, and man, when I got home from work, I couldn't wait to go for my walk. When I returned, the potatoes were gone. The next morning I asked Ken what happened to the potatoes and with complete surprise on his face, he said they were in the carport. He proceeded to look for them in the back of his truck, in the car trunk, went back and forth from the basement several times, and looked in both bedrooms. It was like a whirlwind going by. He opened the door to the living room, and there was the box on the floor. He was stunned and wanted to know who put them there. I told him, "That's O.K., I'm just glad you found them."

Watching him made me so tired. I felt as if I'd already worked all day, and it was still not even daylight. I'm sure it affected him more than me.

09/95

Ken and I went to White Lake which is a family vacation spot. His brother Teddy and his wife Sarah arrived around 1:30 a.m., the following morning. Ken repeatedly questioned them as to what time they arrived.

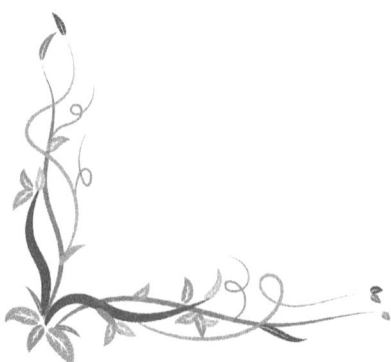

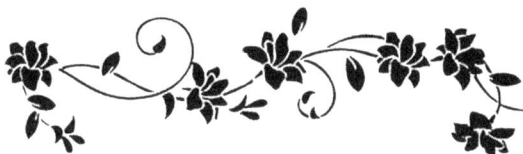

RESTFUL SLEEP

The sun is setting in the west,
and such a beautiful light has been cast.
When we reflect o'er the day just passed
can we lay our head down,
close our eyes and get a good night's rest?
When we met people on the street,
did we smile, or did we speak?
Our thoughts to ourselves did we decide to keep?
Did we share a kind word or deed,
or did we pass someone by,
with no thought to their need?
As we choose the way of life we take,
what type of road do we help make?

09/04/95

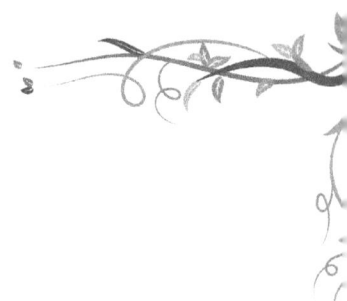

09/07/95

My Dad and I had planned to go to Richmond, Virginia. Ken asked that we not go until he and I returned from White Lake, and that he'd probably go with us. When I asked if he was going with us, he seemed surprised. I then asked, if he wanted me to let him know when we arrived at our destination. He said that would not be necessary. Well, Dad and I left as planned. There were no expressways, with restaurants, no gas pumps on every corner, and no cells.

We traveled several miles on a lonely country road, with not a living creature in sight. All of a sudden there was an awareness—find a bathroom—now!!!! After what seemed like forever, we saw a service station in the distance. The only bathroom was an out-house. It was one of those situations where you either keep riding, hope you can wait; sit over an open space of spiders, and whatever else! (I don't think I'll tell you which I chose.)

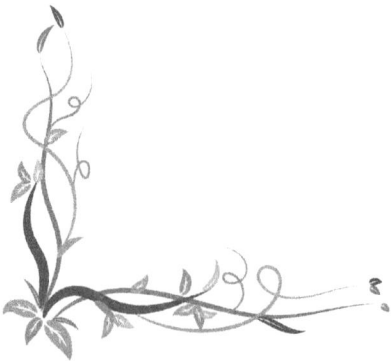

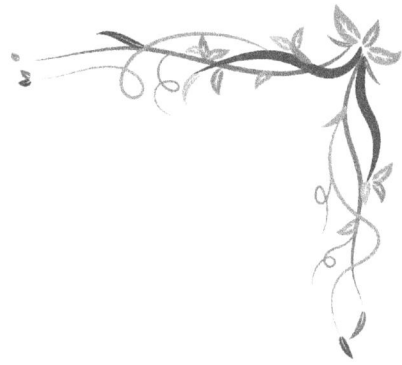

09/08/95

When I came in Friday night, Ken looked at me and didn't say anything, but he seemed puzzled. A neighbor said he had been to visit them while I was gone, and asked several times if they were working Saturday.

09/11/95

I had previously registered in King at one of the banks for a business class offered off campus by Forsyth Tech. I mentioned it to Ken at different times, and when I reminded him today, he did not remember.

09/12/95

I have been seeing Dr. Barbee, a Chiropractor, for my back pains and body adjustments. He advised me to register for a water aerobic exercise. After supper, I reminded Ken that I was going for this, and he hadn't remembered. When I came in tonight, he looked real funny, and said, "Oh, you've been to aerobics. I thought you were helping your Dad pack for his coast trip."

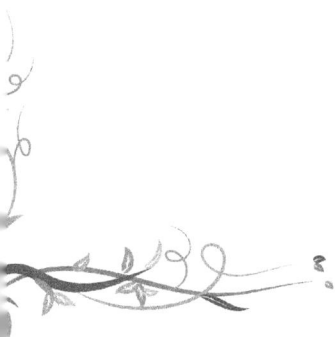

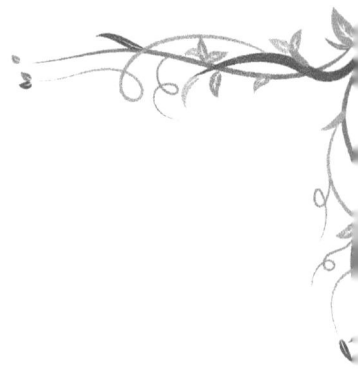

09/13/95

I reminded Ken that I wanted him to meet me at Town & Country Restaurant tomorrow evening to eat before my classes, and then I wouldn't have to drive home and back to King for my classes. He was clueless as to what I was talking about. My life is like walking around the corner, and not knowing what I'll find.

09/14/95

I didn't even mention to Ken to meet me—I know he'll forget. I did remind him about my business class as he was going out the door. His response was, "What class?"

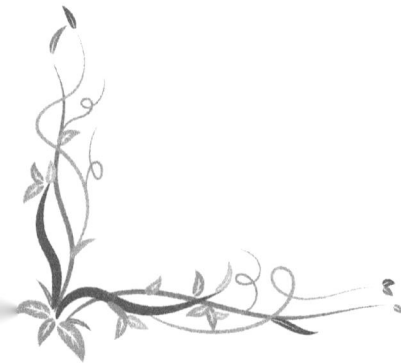

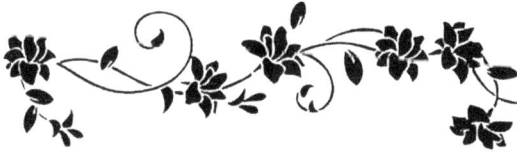

SIMPLE THINGS OF LIFE

Mama, I watched you day by day
as your life on earth slowly slipped away.
I look back with admiration for your concern of the loved ones
you'd be leaving behind.
With no thought of your pain you looked to the future,
and the new life you'd gain.
You'd always enjoyed the simple things of life;
watching the sun come up each morning,
and the squirrels as they played in the trees.
You looked forward to the time when
the fresh green onions would push their way out of the earth.
You enjoyed working in your flowers, and observing the soft summer
showers.
What excitement to gravel for new baby potatoes,
that tasted good enough to serve to the neighbors.
You would chuckle with delight as you watched
the kittens chase the leaves in flight.
No one could sew a dress exactly as you;
a stitch here and a stitch there, and in no time you were through.
The songs that you sang are not sung much anymore,
but in my memory I can hear them once again.
I can still see the smile on your face, Mama
as you talked of your children, your grandchildren,
and your great-grandchildren.
You shared so much of yourself
as you looked to the future and were
content with the simple things of life.

10/06/95

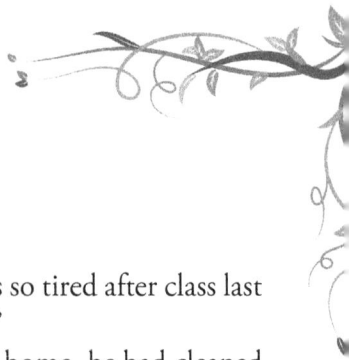

10/10/95

I commented to Ken during supper that I was so tired after class last night. He came back with, "Whose fault is that?"

I had to go to water aerobics, and when I got home, he had cleaned off the table. I thanked him, and as he went outside to smoke, he said, "I'm going to clean it better when I come back in. You're in big trouble. You've done it this time!" I was so bewildered, and racking my brain, as to what I'd done to trigger this type of reaction.

When he finally came back in, he wanted to know what had happened to his warmer work clothes. I explained to him that I have to buy him some new one's, because a couple of uniforms were not wearable. He said, "Don't you ever throw anything of mine away. If you do, I'll go through your closet and burn everything you have! Do you understand me?"

He was so angry with me. I went into the kitchen, so he wouldn't see how he was upsetting me. Almost in the same breath, he asked if my legs had cramped in aerobics, and acted as if he hadn't said, or done anything. Later, he said he had talked to his sister, Alexandria while I was gone. I feel so useless. I know this has to be stressful for Ken, but he won't talk to me about what's going on.

10/29/95

On the way home from church, I asked Ken if he was going to watch the football game. He said that he didn't feel like doing anything, and then he decided to go to Libby Hills Fish Restaurant at Mt. Airy. After eating, he decided to look for a turning plow. We, then stopped at the flea market. On the way home, I asked if he was going to take a nap. He said he was going to see his Mom, and then come back home. This was about 3:00. He didn't come home until 10:00, and I was getting worried.

When he came home, he told me that he had been to see his sister, also. He talked about the visit, and then started fussing at me again, for throwing away his work clothes. The whole time that he was talking, he was rubbing his forehead really hard.

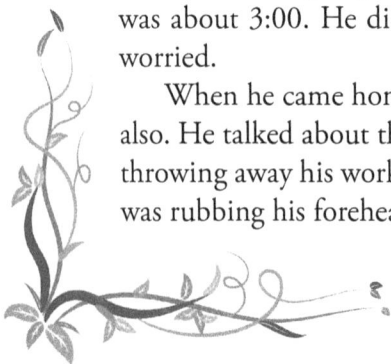

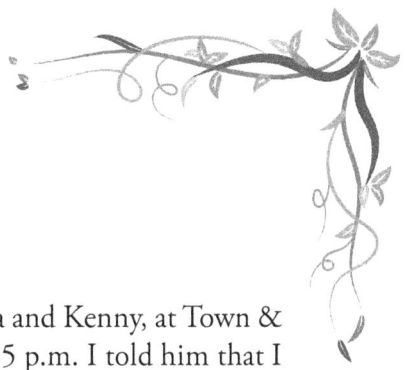

11/04/95

Ken was to meet me and our friends, Donna and Kenny, at Town & Country Restaurant between 6:30 p.m. and 6:45 p.m. I told him that I wasn't sure what time I would be through with my manicure. Traffic on Friday is bad, so I allowed for time. I called Donna just as I was leaving, and she called Ken at 6:25 p.m. to meet us. He didn't answer the phone, so she assumed he was on the way to the restaurant. We waited until 6:50 p.m. and I called him. He said he had already been, he had just got home, and he wasn't coming back! I asked if he had eaten, and he said, "Nope!" I said, "OK." and hung up. I told Donna and Kenny that I was going home.

When I got home, he didn't say anything, and neither did I. I have learned that sometimes it's best to be silent. He just looked at me. After a few minutes, he said, "Did you eat?" I said, "How do you think I could eat knowing you were home and angry, and me not knowing why?" He said, "I didn't speak short to you, I just said, nope." After about an hour, I asked him if he wanted to eat, and he said, "OK." While I was in the kitchen, he came and put his arms around me, kissed me on the cheek and said, "I love you." I don't understand any of this. He ate well, but seemed real withdrawn.

11/06/95

Dad called, and wanted to take us out to lunch. Ken said OK. When we got to the restaurant, Dad, who is 86, had trouble deciding where he wanted to sit. As we were waiting for him to decide, Ken bumped him a little on his shoulder. I began to reprimand him quietly and Daddy shook his head to let it go. I was concerned.

We finally sat down and placed our order for the buffet. Ken waited until Dad & I went to the buffet; came back to the table, and then he went to the buffet. As he got up, he took his hand and pushed against my shoulder three to four times, and then against my face.

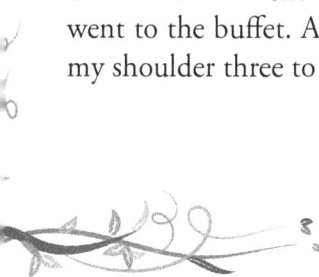

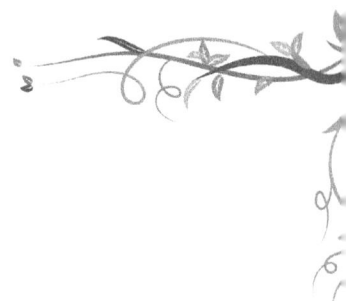

01/03/96

Ken got the adding machine, and sat down at the kitchen table. He kept looking at the calendar, and then at his paycheck stubs. I finally asked him what he was doing. He said he felt he didn't get paid right. I looked at the stubs, and calendar pay periods, and tried to explain to him what I thought they had done. I asked him to wait until tomorrow when he gets paid again, and then if it doesn't look right, to check with payroll. Even then, he kept looking at the calendar, and then back at the paycheck stubs for ever so long. He had such a confused expression on his face. I don't know how to help him.

01/05/96

We played Rook with Donna and Kenny, and Ken played almost as if he had never played before. He made plays that were so unusual for him, and there was a confused look on his face. We tried to help him without him knowing, but I fear a game we have enjoyed playing, is coming to an end.

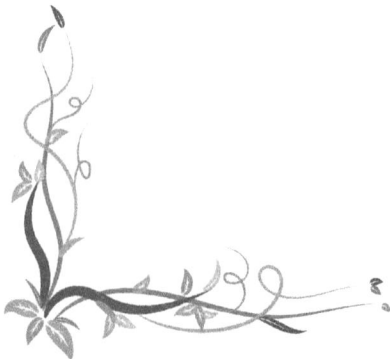

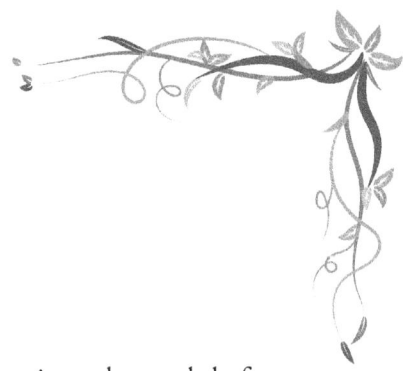

02/23/96

I have been coughing and throwing up a lot since the week before Christmas. I have had tests. Cough syrups and cough drops don't help. When I got home today, I was coughing and gagging, and barely made it to the bathroom. I did this for approximately ½ hour.

As I entered the house, the lights weren't on and Ken was staring at the television. He acted as if he didn't even know that I was sick. Though no fault of his, he probably doesn't remember. As soon as I came out of the bathroom, he stuck out two envelopes and said, "Did you know you had two bills you've not paid?" I was so weak, and out of breath I could hardly answer him. I had paid ½ of the oil bill, and had intended to write a check for the remainder this weekend. I had sent the car payment off, but they didn't post the payment before they sent out a late notice.

Ken was so upset with me. We went out to eat with Donna and Kenny, but he was real restless and couldn't be still, and was still upset with me.

02/24/96

Ken was still withdrawn this morning. I went by to see his Mama while he was there. He looked at me as if to say, what are you doing here? He left almost immediately, and barely spoke to me.

When I got home, we went to the farm. Ken said he wanted to show me the property line. He still seemed as if his mind was elsewhere. He never offered to reach for my hand, nor ask if I needed help in climbing. It was as if he was in his own world.

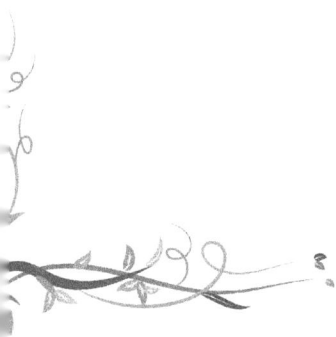

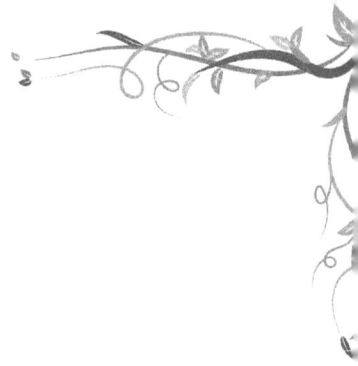

03/03/96

I wasn't feeling well, and my head was sort of floating. I took a capsule that Dr. McGuirt had prescribed, and went back to bed. Ken went to church. I had lunch ready when he came home. His back was hurting, and he seemed restless. He left, and I assumed he had gone to see his Mom. When he came home, he said he had been to Alexandria's, but that she wasn't home. I then asked if he went to Teddy's, and he said "Yes." He later tried to call Alexandria. Our phone has been out of order since the ice storm. He became real agitated, walked by me, reached out and flipped his fingers against my breast. He later walked by me, balled up his fist, and said, "Don't say a word to me." I just looked at him, and then he smiled, and hugged me.

03/11/96

I called the telephone company, and supposedly it was our cordless phone. Ken wanted to make a long distance call, and started working on the main phone, then the cordless phone. I was sick, and wanted to go to bed. Usually, Ken is ready for bed at 8:00, but tonight he kept fooling with the phone, and finally walked out to Gail's. We have no problem with local calls. Later, when I said, "I'm calling Daddy," he wanted to know how I could call him, when the phone doesn't work. He fooled with phone for about two hours.

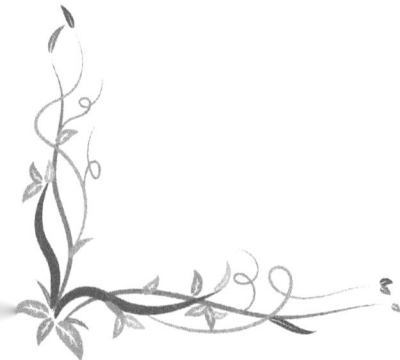

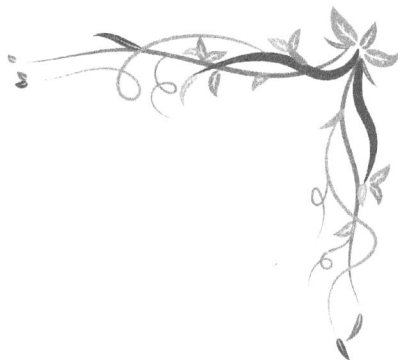

03/12/96

I came in from work, and then went to see Dr. Barbee. I was only gone about one hour. When I came in Ken was in his solitude mood. He barely spoke, and seemed withdrawn. He said he had called Dobson, and the lady said there was nothing wrong with phone. He said he called the same number, and got Rocky Mount. I questioned him, but he was positive he had dialed the same number, but couldn't remember what number he had dialed.

03/14/96

Gail said after she had talked to Ken the other night, she wanted to talk to me. She had asked Ken the same question three times. She couldn't get him to understand and didn't dare to say anything to him. I was in the kitchen, and had turned around to walk to the den, when Ken came from that direction. He had been working on the cordless phone again. As he came around the corner, he still had the screwdriver in his hand. He stuck it right at my stomach, and laughed, and said "I bet you lost two pounds. Wasn't that easy?"

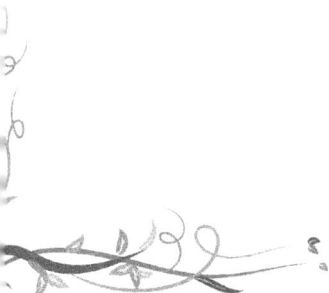

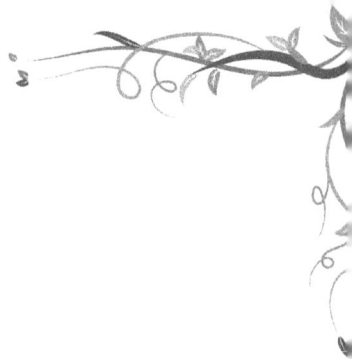

03/18/96

Ken's brother, Teddy, called and told me they want to have a birthday dinner for their mother on 04/14/96 after church. He then talked to Ken. He told Ken when they were planning on the dinner, and how old she'd be, etc. Ken thought she was 86 or 87. Before he hung up, he said, "I know how old she is, and laughed." He then called a cousin, and during the conversation said, "We're having a birthday dinner for Mama on Sunday after church. I'm not sure how old she will be. I think 66 or 67."

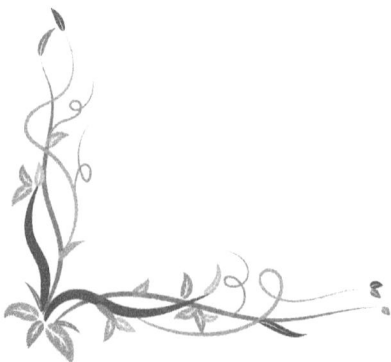

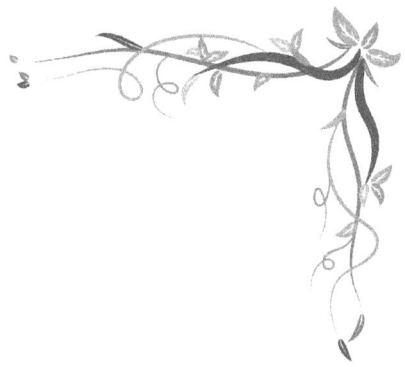

03/30/96

I had purchased a used typewriter, and wanted to run an extension cord in the basement from an outlet. Ken said no, that he would run a wire for a plug-in. I asked him to get an electrician, or someone to help, and he asked, "Don't you think I know how?" I said "Yes, I know you do, but wouldn't it be easier to have someone else to do it?" I know at one time, he could have done this with no problem, but I'm uncomfortable with this. He left about 9:00 a.m. to go get what he needed. I left at same time.

When I got home approximately at 1:00 p.m., Ken was in the basement. I heard Ken making a lot of noise. Ken, then came upstairs. When he began pulling out drawers, I asked, "what are you looking for? " He wanted to know where the wire cutters were. I had no idea. I named several places they might be, but he had already looked.

He then went back to the basement, and about 2:00 p.m. came back up, and said "I've done all that I'm doing today. All I lack is hooking up to the box." I said "OK., why don't you rest awhile?" He said he didn't have time, but eventually he did sit down for a few minutes. He said "I want to wait 'til I'm by myself to finish. I said, "There's no one here but me, and I'm not bothering you." He said" I want to be by myself, so I can think when I connect the wire. It's taken me all day to do a 45 minute job."

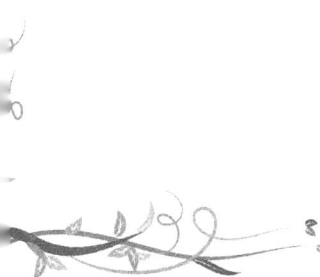

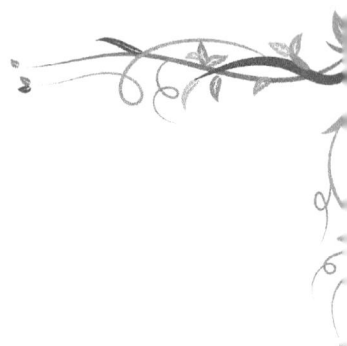

04/06/96

Ken left at 7:00 a.m. before I got up, and came in about 10:00 a.m. He had been out to eat breakfast, and then went to see his sister, Alexandria. He sat down in his recliner, and seemed real restless all day. Later in the evening he said his head was hurting, and went to bed at 8:00 p.m.

04/08/96

I worked until 5:15 p.m. and when I got home, Ken was watching T.V. with no lights on. He gave me a real hard look when I walked in, and turned back to the T.V. without speaking. I asked, "Why are you sitting in the dark?" He said, "I'm watching T.V. and I don't need lights." All of the lights are usually on. He was real withdrawn and uncommunicative.

04/09/96

Ken, started looking again for his wire cutter. He found it beside his chair in the paper stand. He then turned toward me, and clipped at my nose several times. I backed away from him. He laughed and hugged me and said, "I wouldn't hurt you for anything. I was picking on you." My nerves are working overtime.

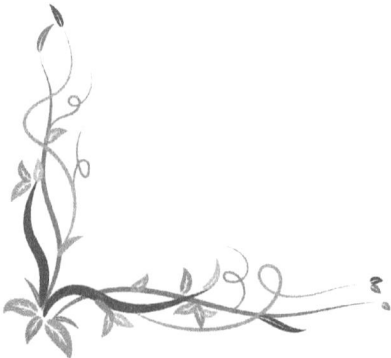

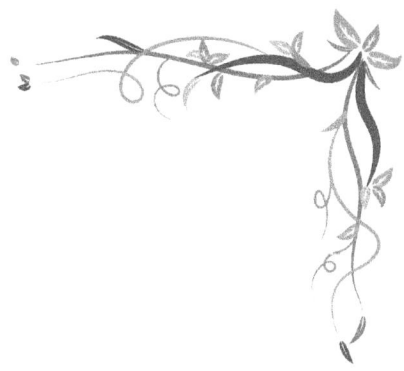

04/11/96

As I was cooking supper, Ken came in the kitchen, and put his arms around me. He seemed to be in a loving mood.

Ken decided to take a bath, and I decided to play the piano for relaxation. As I was playing the piano, he asked me where his older work shirts were. He then, wanted to know if I had thrown away any of his shirts? I told him no. He asked," Are you sure? Where are they? Why don't I have any to match this pair of pants?" I told him, "I'm tired of you continuing to bring that back up, and I don't want to hear it anymore!"

I continued playing the piano as Ken went in the den, and sat down in his recliner. He didn't turn on the T.V. but stared straight ahead without moving. I went to the bathroom to take my shower, and before I began, a friend called. He brought the phone to me. He was real friendly to her, but gave me one of his looks before closing the door. He was in bed when I came out.

04/12/96

Ken came to tell me bye before he left for work this morning. I had just awakened. He said, "You know you're beautiful, but life plays funny tricks." I'm not sure what he meant.

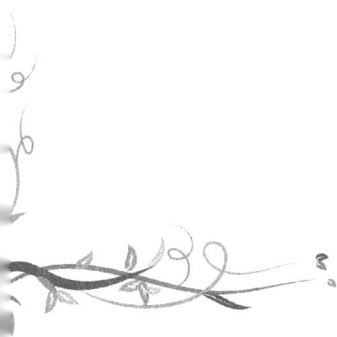

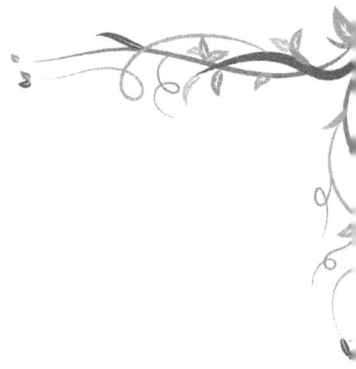

04/13/96

I asked Ken about something I had seen in the storage building when I went to get my flower sprinkler. He said, "So you are the one who left the door open. I closed it Friday." I said, "I left it open Saturday. Did you go down there yesterday?" He said, "You couldn't have left it open Saturday, 'cause I closed it Friday." When we got home, I went in the house. He came in a little later, and said, "I told you I closed it Friday." I feel like a goldfish swimming around in circles.

04/16/96

When I came in from work, Ken was in his recliner holding his hands on each side of his head, which he does so often. I asked him if he was alright, and he said "yes." He came into the kitchen and said, "I think I'll go to bed. I'm sleepy, and my head hurts." He ate, and then went to bed about 9:00.

04/19/96

We went out to eat, and Ken seemed confused when he was ordering his food. When given a choice of a baked potato or French fries, and butter or sour cream, etc. he had a confused expression on his face.

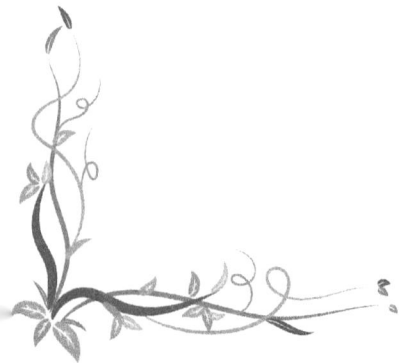

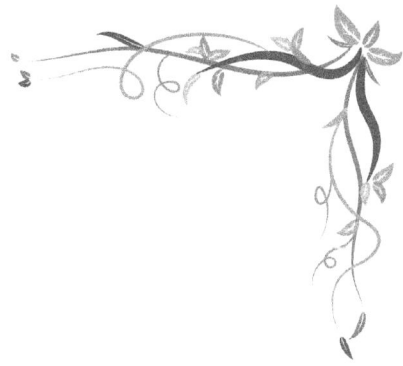

04/20/96

We went out again to eat with friends, and Ken had no idea what he wanted. He has done this so often. He will look at the menu as if he really isn't seeing what is there. He has new glasses, so I don't think that's it.

05/18/96

I talked with Dr. Roach about Ken's symptoms, and he said he definitely needs treatment.

I tried to get Ken to go see Dr. Roach, but he wouldn't, so I asked his brother to talk with him.

06/05/96

Ken finally went to see Dr. Roach, who talked with him and asked him questions. Ken then had his blood drawn. When the doctor went out of the room, Ken looked at me and said, "I know what you're going to do." I asked him, "What?" He said, "You're going to have me committed, sell everything we have, and marry a black man." I don't know where that came from.

Dr. Roach wrote a prescription for Cognex, and within two weeks I can tell he's calmer. Ken had blood work, MRI, EKG, EEG's. For a period of time, it seemed that we lived in medical offices.

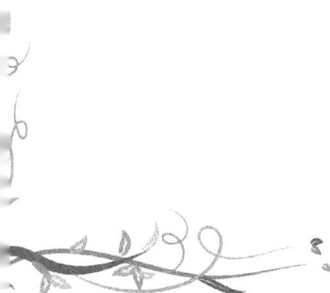

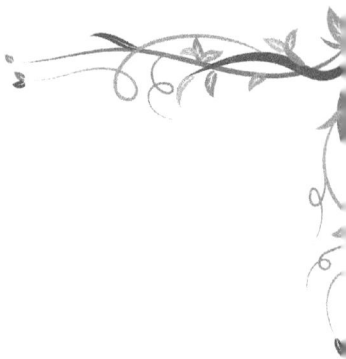

06/15/96

Ken umpired behind the plate for two softball games. He came home, took a shower, and said he was going to see his Mama. He left, and I started to Daddy's and met Ken. I turned around, and followed him home. He was hosing off the truck tires that were covered with mud. He seemed rather shaken. I said, "I thought you were going to see your mom." He said, "No, I went to the farm." I have no idea what had happened. He went in the house, and I told him that I was going to check on Daddy, and would cook supper when I got back. He said "OK., and then we'll go see Mama." He still seemed shaken when I returned from Dad's, but he ate a good supper.

06/16/96

Ken went to bed early last night, and got up about 7:00 this morning after sleeping good all night. He then lay on the couch, and went back to sleep. He has slept almost all day, and admitted that he doesn't feel good.

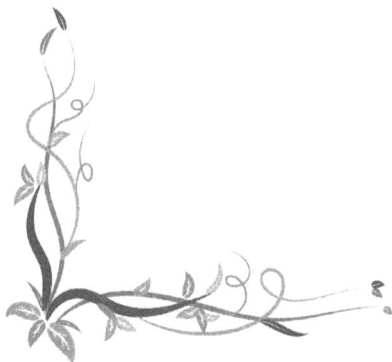

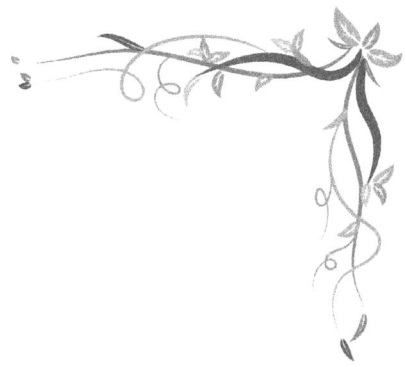

06/17/96

When I got home from work, my niece called and asked if I could stay with my brother, for a couple of hours. He had a tooth cut out, and couldn't be left alone. Ken said, "Go on, and don't worry about supper."

When I got home at 8:45, he was lying on the couch with his head on the arm rest, and rolling it back and forth. He was rubbing the top and temple of his head. He told me that he had taken Tylenol. He seemed to be in so much pain. I asked him if it hurt like when his sinuses bothered him, and he said, "No, so much pressure." I don't have any idea what is going on with him. He wouldn't go to the emergency room. He went to bed, and slept restless all night.

06/18/96

Ken didn't remember me going to my brother's, my coming home, nor him having the headache. He was real tired this morning.

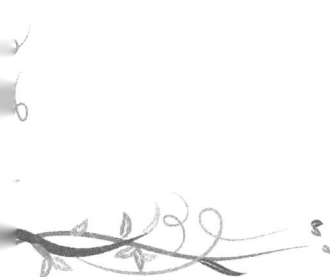

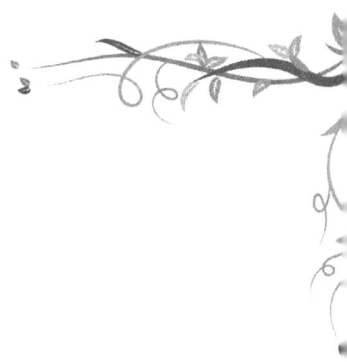

06/22/96

Ken got up early, and went out for breakfast. He came home, and said he was going to Belews Creek to see his Aunt Joanie, whom he hasn't seen in years. I asked him to wait until I got back home, and I'd go with him. He said, "No." He came home about 12:30, and looked as if he could hardly walk through the door. He said, "I'm give out." I wish I knew how to help him. He slept off and on all evening.

06/23/96

Ken got up, and I could tell he didn't feel good. We went to church, but when we came home he lay down, and slept until 2:30.

06/30/96

We went to church, and stayed for homecoming. When we got home, he lay down, and slept a couple of hours.

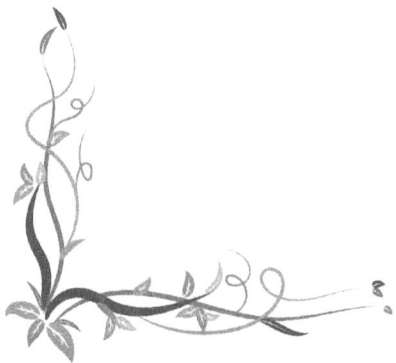

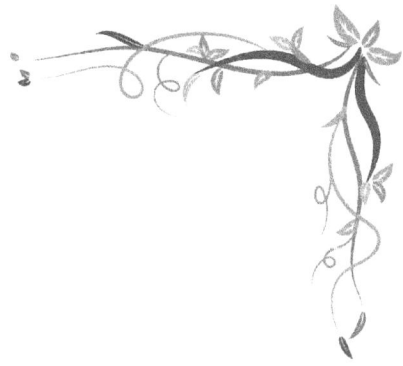

07/04/96

Ken got up early, and went out to eat breakfast. We went to Wytheville, Virginia, and had lunch. When we came back, he played golf with friends. He seemed tired, but content, and said he had played good.

07/05/96

Ken said he had gone to the farm and cleaned off some creek banks. He seemed to be alright. I'm not sure why he thinks the creek banks need cleaning off, but I've learned not to say anything to him.

07/06/96

Ken played golf today. When he came in, he said, "You can sell these clubs at your next yard sale. I'm hanging it up. I played terrible." He took the clubs to the basement. Later, when I talked with his friends, they told me that he had thrown his clubs, and kept hitting the balls into the water.

07/12/96

Ken had a lumbar puncture today which he tolerated well. He slept part of the day, and lay on the couch or in his recliner, when not in bed. He said the pressure was not as bad since the fluid was withdrawn.

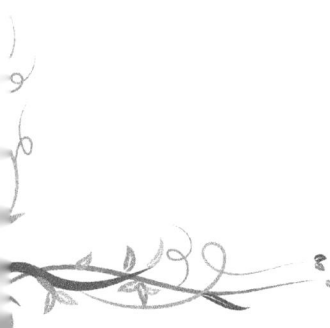

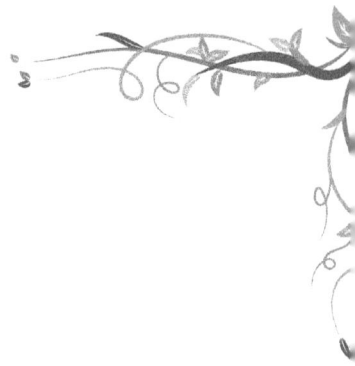

07/27/96

Ken went out to eat breakfast. I went to the garden to pick green beans to can. When I returned, Ken was in his recliner, and appeared withdrawn. Dad came to help me string the beans. Ken came outside and began helping.

We had planned to go to a wedding, and I told him that we could stop, and get ready. He said he didn't feel like it, that he was as nervous as a cat on a hot tin roof. I noticed that his hands were shaking. He went inside, and slept for a couple of hours.

Ken then got up, and said, "I'm going to see Mama." I asked him if I called the restaurant for a take-out, would he pick it up for me and Dad. He said, "No, I'm going to see Mama." He came home about 7:00 p.m., and was still restless. He finally went to sleep about 12:00 a.m.

07/28/96

Ken was up before me. We went to church, but I could tell he wasn't feeling good. During worship service, he kept rubbing his head. We went out to eat with a couple from church. When we got home, we both went to sleep. When I woke up, he was gone. When he came home, he said he had been to see his Mama, but seemed confused.

07/29/96

Ken may have slept three hours last night. He was very restless, and was up and down, tossing and turning all night.

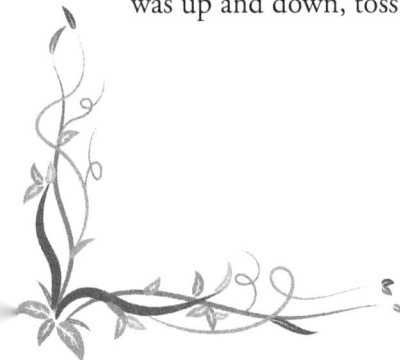

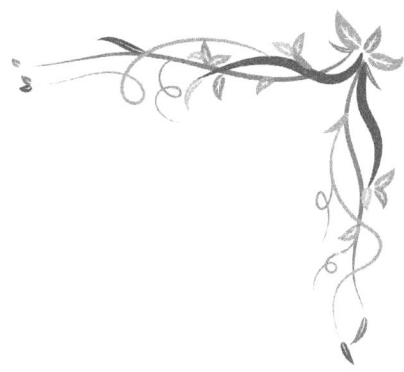

08/03/96

Ken has not slept well for several days, and has been real restless.

08/04/96

We didn't go to church today. I was up until 1:30 a.m. canning green beans, and I wasn't feeling well. Ken didn't rest well, and said his back was hurting, and didn't feel like going. Later today, he said, "I'm not taking any more of my medicine, 'cause the doctor doesn't know what's wrong with me anyway." He did finally take it.

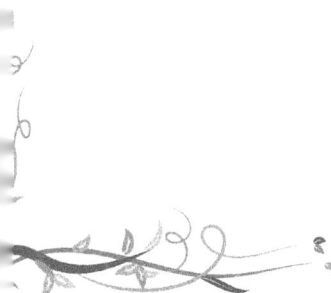

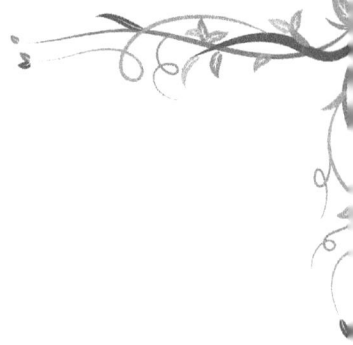

8/05/96

We got up early this morning. Ken was scheduled for his second spinal tap for pressure. He was in a bad mood, and barely spoke. He usually stops at Bojangles for breakfast. I asked if he wanted to stop and he said, "I'm not hungry." I, then said, "You need to at least get a cup of coffee, and take your medicine." His reply was, "I've already had a cup of coffee, and I'm not taking my medicine."

He was extremely restless while waiting at the hospital. He finally said, "I'm going to smoke a cigarette." I told him that he needed to check at the desk because they may be ready for him. He said, "I've waited on them, and they can wait on me." I did ask, and they said he had time.

When they completed the test, he was supposed to ride in a wheelchair to the pick-up zone. He refused, but could hardly walk out of the hospital. He wanted a cup of coffee, so I went to the cafeteria to get one for him. I, then told him to wait while I went to get the car. He refused, and said "I reckon I can walk." He wouldn't lay the seat back, and refused to fasten his seat belt.

When we got home, he went across the road, and talked to Frank for approximately thirty minutes. He came in, ate something, and after about two hours, he laid down. He was in a terrible mood all day. His brother and sister-in-law came, and he went outside so they could smoke.

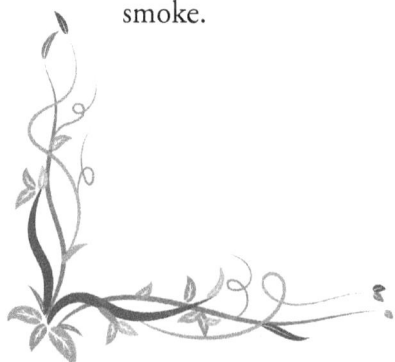

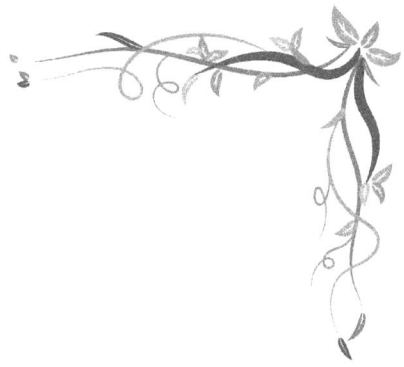

08/06/96

Ken slept very little last night. When he went to the bathroom, he could hardly walk. He didn't work today, and he needed to stay at home.

08/07/96-08/09/96

Ken hasn't slept well all week. He has worked, has had really bad headaches, and gone to bed about 8:00 p.m.

08/10/96

We went to Lowe's Hardware for some florescent lights and ballasts. When we came back, Ken worked on those. I asked him to wait because I knew he didn't feel well. I trimmed bushes, and then he tried to help me. I told him not to, but he did anyway. He looks terrible, and doesn't feel well at all.

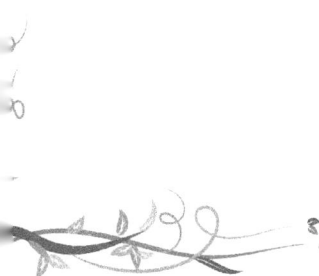

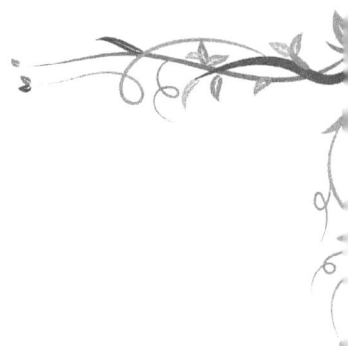

08/11/96

We went to church and Ken kept rubbing his head and temples. After we ate lunch, he went to bed and slept for a couple of hours. When he woke up, he went to see his Mom.

08/14/96

As we were eating supper, Clark came to spray for bugs, as he does on a regular basis. He said "Go ahead and eat, and I'll spray outside." We finished eating, and I cleaned up the dishes. I gathered my bowls, knife, and brush, ready to go to the garden, to pull and shuck corn.

It's corn shucking and freezing time. In preparation, I had already put buckets and my pocketbook, in the truck. I came back in to change clothes, and then went to the kitchen. I was between the table and refrigerator, as Ken came in from outside. As I moved to give him room to come in, he went by me and he said, "Take good care of the corn." As Ken spoked laughingly, he put his hand flat against my back, between my shoulder blades. He pushed me real hard toward the storm door.

I lost my balance, but was able to keep from falling, as I went on out the door onto the carport. Clark just stood there with his mouth open. He had never seen Ken like this. My garden shoes were beside the steps. I hurriedly put them on, and as I was tying them, Ken came out the door and said, "I'm sorry." I told him he should be, and got in the truck. I was shaking like a leaf, and I forgot my bowls.

When I got back home at 8:45, Ken was in the bed. The phone rang as I was getting in the shower. When I answered, it was Delight, Ken's sister, and she wanted to speak to him. I told her that he was probably asleep, and I'd rather not wake him.

She still insisted that she talk to her brother. She had nothing to say to me. I woke him up, and took my shower.

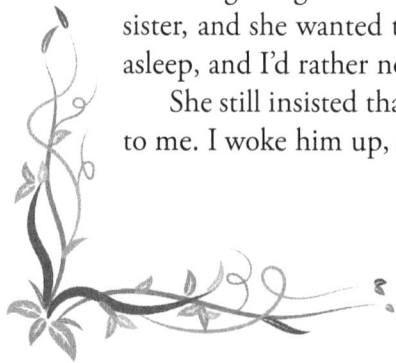

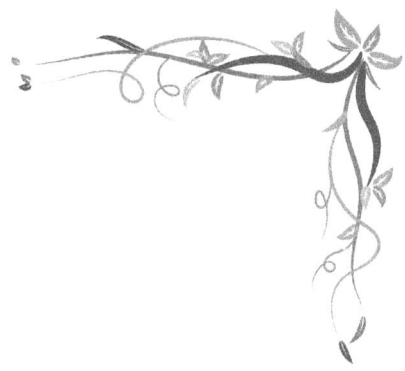

08/15/96

Ken came to the bedroom this morning to tell me bye before he went to work. He acted as if nothing had happened last night. He probably didn't remember.

8/20/96

Ken said this morning that he was going to the farm after work today, and push up some trees. I said, "You don't want to eat at Town & Country?" He said, "No, I'm going to the farm." I said, "OK. then I won't come home after work, because I need to use Donna's computer. I'll get a bite to eat, and bring you something." I changed my mind. I went by the dry cleaners at King, and as I was getting on 52 North, I saw Ken exiting 52 South. I went on to the bank, changed my clothes, and went back to Town & Country.

Ken was sitting outside looking down at his hands. I said, "It's a good thing I saw you 'cause I hadn't planned to eat here. What made you change your mind?" He said, "I just did." I don't know if he remembered what he told me this morning. It's confusing for me, also.

08/27/96

Dr. Crowell took Ken off Cognex because his enzyme level was four times too high. Ken said he didn't like to take them as they slowed him down. He is still having real bad headaches.

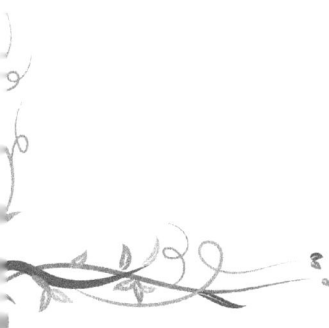

08/30/96

We left this morning for Florida with Teddy and Sarah. Ken was real quiet. He looked at the scenery as we rode, and slept some. I had taken monies out of our savings, and gave him half. I told him that I would put my half in the safe in our room. When we needed it, we could get it. When we checked out, we would use the cash not spent to pay on room rate, and put balance on our Visa.

Ken asked me every day if I had paid for our room. Each time, I explained to him. We went to Silver Springs, Kennedy Space Center, Sea World, and Cypress Garden. Naturally, we did a lot of walking. He would go one direction, as we went another. We were forever calling for him to come where we were. He seemed to intentionally stay by himself. Some things he refused to do, and would say. "Go ahead, I'll wait," but we wouldn't go off and leave him.

He and Teddy played golf on Thursday afternoon. Sarah had already told me that Teddy wanted to treat Ken, and that he wouldn't take any money for the game. Later that night, Ken said, "I need to pay Teddy for the golf game." I sat there for a moment before I said anything. Then I said, "Sometimes you have to let people do things for you, just because they want to." He didn't say anything else about it.

When we left Friday morning, I asked Ken how much cash he had left, and he said, "What do you want to know for?" I explained to him again, and it seemed he just couldn't understand. I knew he had at least $100.00, so I paid my cash toward the room.

On the way home, we stopped at a place that sold fruit, and I asked for some money to get oranges, and he almost didn't give it to me. I gave him back approximately $80.00. We stopped at the Cracker Barrel in Concord to eat supper.

A cousin and his wife were also there, whom I usually see once a year. As we finished eating, I commented that I wanted to speak to him while we waited on the ticket. Ken stood up, and said very loudly, "Hold on a minute. I've paid for everything since we've been gone. It's time you paid for something!" I said, "Ken, you have the money." He said, "No, I don't, you didn't give it back to me!" I said, "Yes, I did." He said, "I reckon I know; you didn't give it to me." I said, "Ken, look in your billfold, you do have the money." He looked and said real softly,

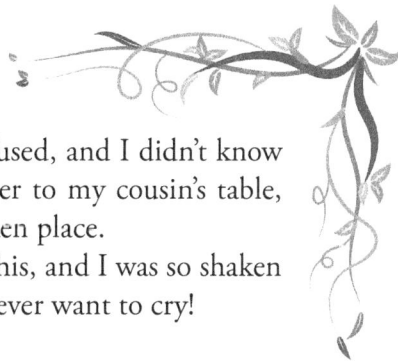

"OK." and sat back down. I knew he was confused, and I didn't know what to do. In about five minutes he came over to my cousin's table, shook his hand, and acted as if nothing had taken place.

I felt as if everyone in the room witnessed this, and I was so shaken by it. I never raised my voice to him, but did I ever want to cry!

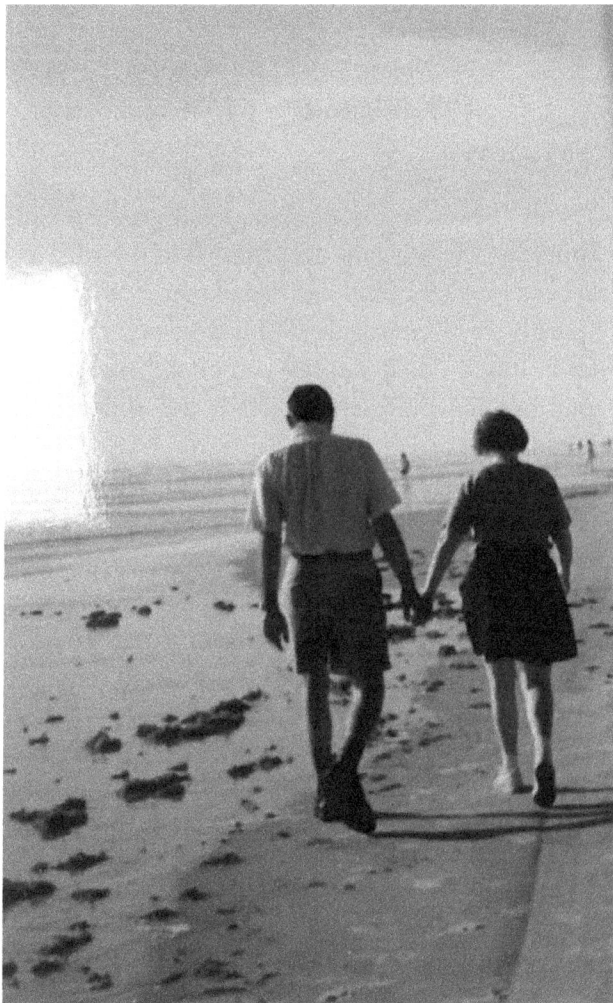

Ken and Polly strolling on the beach in Florida in August 1996

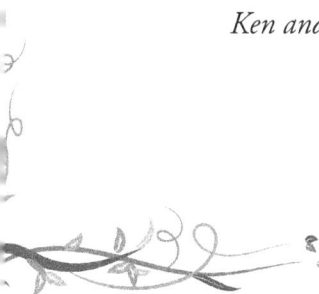

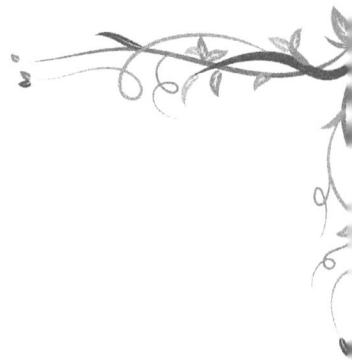

09/07/96-09/14/96

Ken has hardly spoken to me all week. I was on the telephone when he came in Thursday. He was late, and I didn't know where he was. He gave me a real hard look. A friend had called who needed to talk. When I got off the telephone, Ken asked, "Who were you talking to?" I told him, and then he asked. "Did she call you or did you call her?" I said, "She called me, but it wouldn't have made any difference." He said, "Oh, yes it would have, too."

Saturday, Ken left early and went to the farm. I had an appointment to get my hair cut at 5:00 P.M. I had everything ready except finalizing supper, if he wanted to eat at home. He came in as I was leaving. I asked if he wanted to meet me at Town & Country, or eat at home. He said, "I'm not meeting you anywhere. You do your thing, and I'll do mine. I've got a debt to pay." I stood there with a puzzled look, and he said, "Don't act like you don't know what I'm talking about." I said, "I don't." He said, "I owe Teddy for that golf game. I said, "I don't care if you pay him." He said, "Well, you acted like it made you mad, when I said I wanted to pay him." This is what had been bothering him.

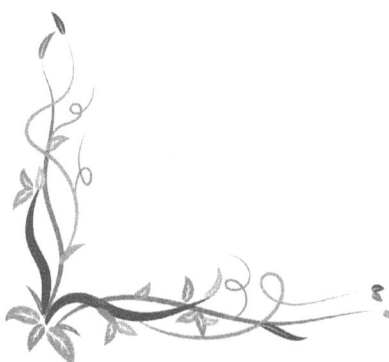

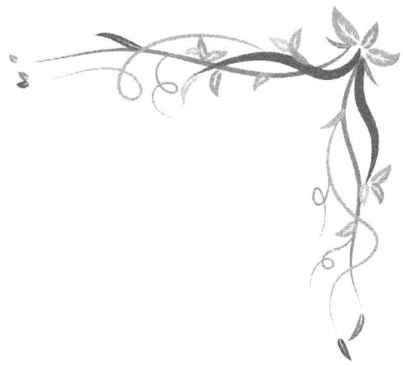

09/22/96

Ken went to a former church for a special service. I didn't go because I wasn't feeling well. When he came home, he acted as if he had a good time, and named several people he had seen. No indication that anything is wrong at all with his memory.

09/24/96

We received a call last night at approximately 9:15 P.M. that Ken's mother was being taken to Forsyth Hospital. I had to wake him up. We didn't get home and in bed until 2:00 A.M.

Ken was sitting beside me, when I called his employer, to notify them of his Mom's death. Employees are allowed time off for deaths of parents. Five minutes later he said, "Did you call work for me?" I wrote my phone number at work for him to call me, and he put it in his shirt pocket. Just before I left, he said, "Was you going to give me your phone number?"

09/26/96

Ken remembered this afternoon that I had planned to go to my nephew's football game. What is so confusing is that his sister said as she was introducing him to someone today, he just walked off.

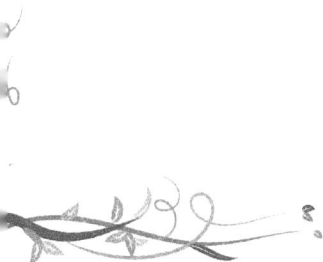

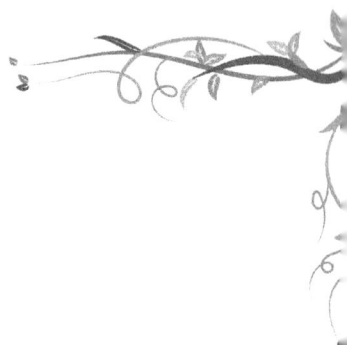

09/27/96

Before I left this morning, I wrote a note for Ken to put in his shirt pocket to meet me at Town & Country at 6:30 P.M. He said he wasn't working today, and was going to see his Mama. He never called me, so I assumed she was doing about the same.

I arrived at Town & Country at 6:30 P.M., and waited until 6:50 P.M., and no Ken. The cashier said that he hadn't been there. I went home and every light in the house was on, and Ken was in the basement. He had drawers pulled out all over the house. He said he was looking for his glasses. I said, "Where do you remember having them?" He said, "I don't know, I can't remember."

Ken had been to the farm, so we went to the farm to look. He had been using the tractor to push up trees. I figured he took them off, and put in his shirt pocket, and they fell out. We never found them. (I bought him a new pair, but he was constantly taking them off, putting in his shirt pocket, or laying them down.)

09/28/96

Ken was up early this morning, but lay back down on the couch and went back to sleep. When he woke up, he didn't want any coffee, and said he was going to look for his glasses. I went over later, and he was back on the tractor pushing trees and debris toward the creek bank.

Ken would put the tractor in reverse, and almost as quickly go forward, and make the tractor stand up. It was so hard to watch him. As Dad and I were watching him I commented, "Why is he pushing the trees toward the creek?" Dad said, "I wondered the same, but didn't say anything to him. He acts as if he's trying to deal with something that's bothering him." Dad told me to go on home, and he'd stay, so Ken wouldn't be by himself. Ken was like a man being driven by a demon.

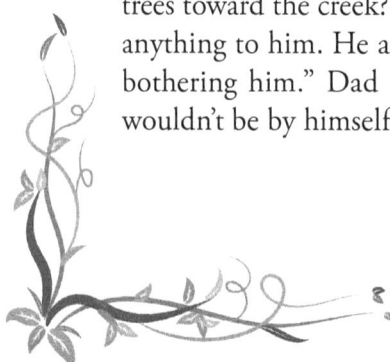

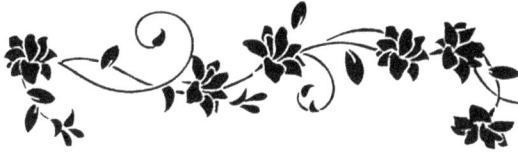

EVELYN

I sit here watching you sleep
as your life is slowly leaving.
So many decisions to be made,
and no one knows which the right one is.
Only God knows when your last breath will come.
Family gathers around to offer what
love and comfort they can.
It hurts them as they hear
you cry out in pain.
We watch, and wait, not knowing
when your time on earth will end.
We have peace in our heart
knowing that when you
Take your last breath,
Sweet heaven you'll see.

10/03/96

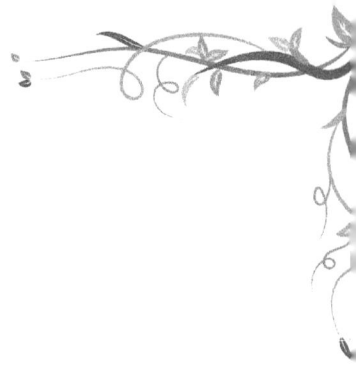

10/04/96

I stopped to get gas on my way home, and Ken drove by, turned around and came back. He said, "Why didn't you answer your phone at work? I left you a message to meet me at Town & Country. I called twice at 3:30 P.M. and whoever answered hung up on me." I don't know who he called, but I didn't have a message. Ken left his truck, and we went on to the hospital to see his Mama. He kept telling me to drive further down to find a better parking space. He kept hollering at me, and finally grabbed the steering wheel, and said, "I said turn to the left. Do you want me to drive?"

When I finally found a space, I couldn't park to suit him. He started yelling at me again. I was so nervous and shaking all over, but couldn't let him know this. When we were around the rest of the family, I had to act as if everything was alright. They were already of the opinion that whatever was wrong with Ken was my fault.

10/05/96-10/07/96

He has seemed to be so aloof from me. It's as if he has no need for me at all. When he's around his family, he doesn't seem to want me around. His mother passed away while in the hospital. The night of the viewing, I put Ken's clothes together, and he dressed. He couldn't remember how to tie his necktie, and became so frustrated. (At the time, I didn't know how, but I did learn.) When we got to the funeral home, he had to ask someone to help him. They thought he was kidding.

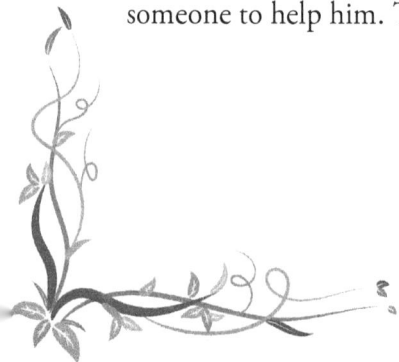

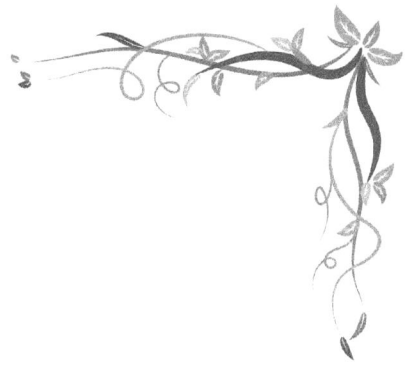

10/96-10/97

(Things have happened this year that were too painful to write about. I've had to do a lot of soul searching, and a lot of praying in order to survive. I am held accountable for how I handle situations. I can't answer for what others do, or don't do.)

Writing poems and putting words on paper is my way of coping life's challenges and serves as a testimony on that certain moment. It was as if an inner being was pushing to be heard, and to remember, I had to write it down.

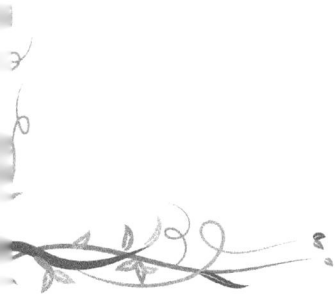

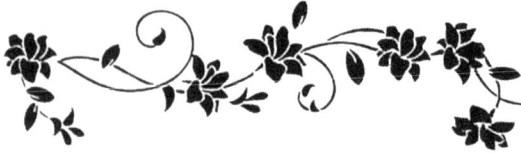

BUILDING DREAMS

In a moment of anger he spoke harshly to her
never realizing how detrimental he had been.
Words can be constructive,
or words can destroy.
As each day progresses, words of encouragement
are needed so much more.
Children can have their dreams
smothered before they take root and grow;
and then adults wonder
why their children have nothing significant to show.
We should build up, not tear down,
another person's feelings.
The Bible teaches us that
young men will dream dreams,
and old men will have visions.
Both are inevitable
as we live each day of our lives.

01/29/96

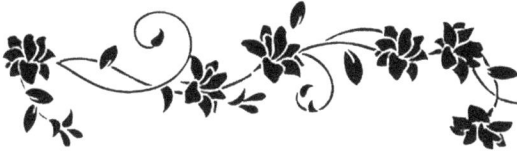

I SAW AN OLD MAN

I saw an old man with a long white beard
shuffling as he walked along the street.
His clothes were worn and shabby,
as they covered his feeble body.
I wonder what experiences he could have shared
and if old age had crept up
and caught him unaware.
So much wisdom he may could
have passed on to me,
but all I could do was pass him by, and bid him God-Speed.
It was such a beautiful warm day
as I saw an old man shuffling
along the way.

03/23/96

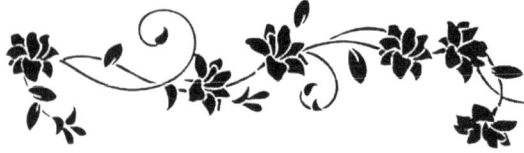

WIND SONGS IN THE NIGHT

There is a whispering sound
as the breeze softly traces
a path thru the grass and leaves.
The sky is ablaze with stars lighting up the night.
Soft furry creatures scatter thru the forest.
Night sounds change as the breeze
picks up the leaves,
and places them so intricately in another location.
The wind chimes come alive with music
as the puff of air playfully moves
through the different shapes.
There is a hushed sound as in the dark of night
the owl lets everyone know that he
is alert as he hunts for food.
The momentum seems to increase as it brings the
sounds of the frogs and crickets,
and lays them at your feet.
Night sounds can sometimes be frightening
but, when you listen close enough,
you can hear the
beautiful wind songs in the night.

04/01/96

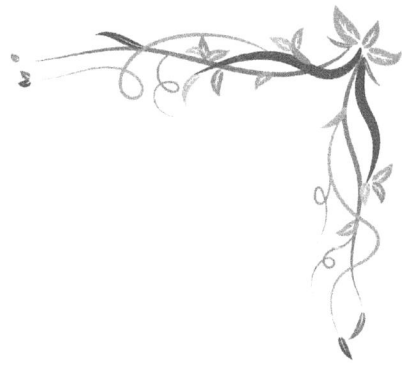

I wrote the following poem about a young man who was a slow learner, but some of his paintings have sold for thousands of dollars.

HIDDEN IMPRESSIONS

They laughed at me 'cause I was different.
They laughed at me 'cause I didn't grasp
things that came to them so naturally.
My impressions were painted in pictures
that sometimes portrayed a mixture of thoughts.
There were images of present and future
that unfolded collectively
as if sewn together with sutures.
People would talk as if I had no knowledge to share.
I would become so frustrated when they couldn't realize
that I had so much to offer,
and it was there displayed
right in front of their eyes.

05/03/96

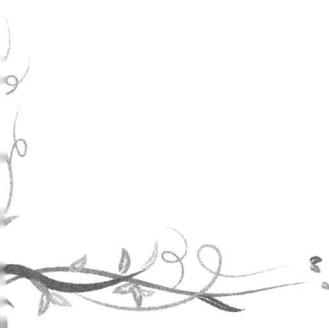

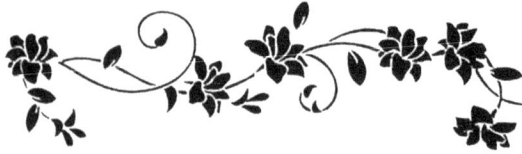

LITTLE CHILDREN

Lightning flashes and thunder rumbles
as rain beats against the window pane.
The drops of rain makes everything
fresh and like new again.
As the sun comes out, the droplets glisten
on the blades of grass.
The flower petals reach out to the moisture
that sustains its' beauty.
The birds bathe in the birdbath,
and sing as if given new life.
Little children play in the mud puddles
with mud squishing between their toes.
They have no thought of life tomorrow,
nor what may follow.
Their laughter is so catching,
and their smiles ever so fetching.

08/22/96

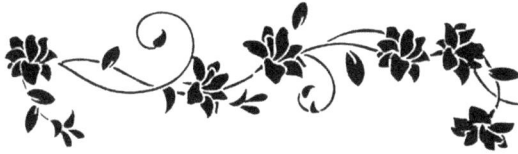

DECISIONS AND CHOICES

I kicked a small rock
to see how far it would go.
It rolled and bounced as it tossed to and fro.
Rocks come in different sizes and shapes;
so do people.
A rock has no choice as to where it will go.
It follows the path of least resistance.
We, as humans, do have a choice,
and it's up to us as to which
path we take.
We have to live with the
decisions and choices we make.

08/12/96

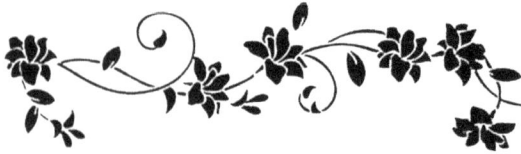

A BUTTERFLY'S KISS

A butterfly kissed me on my shoulder,
and then it flew away
to brighten someone else's day!
The resplendent blue embroidered
with threads of black and yellow
are indescribable.
It's so hard to comprehend
how something that crawls,
and is ugly,
can go through such a metamorphic change.
It's a wonder of wonders
to watch as the worm
turns into such a beautiful piece of art,
not made by hand.

08/19/96

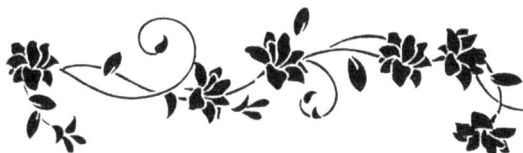

WHERE WILL YOU HIDE

You have such a confused look in your eyes again.
You don't remember where you're going,
and you don't know where you've been.
Your thoughts have taken you so far away.
I often wonder what went wrong.
What happened to the person I once knew.
You've hidden inside your shell for so long,
I'm not sure which is the real you.
A turtle hides in its shell,
and only comes out when it feels safe,
and all is well.
You isolate your feelings, and hold them inside.
A certain part of your past, you continue to hide.
There'll come a time when those emotions will break
as the breaking of a tide.
Where will you turn?
Where will you hide?

10/03/96

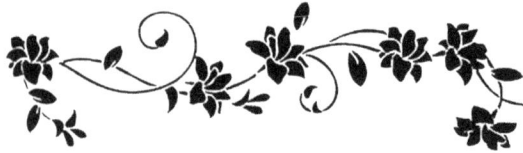

ROWING ALONE

The rain falls, and the wind blows,
and sometime problems that confront us
seem so overwhelming.
We can't decide what to do or
which direction to go.
There comes a time when we have to sit back,
and just go with the flow.
A canoe needs two oars rowing together
in order to ride through the waters smoothly.
If only one oar is used, it makes for a rough ride.
This is true in life.
Whatever the reason may be,
when one person is rowing alone,
he or she should never lose sight
of the beauty in a rainbow,
and the treasures that it bestows.

10/10/96

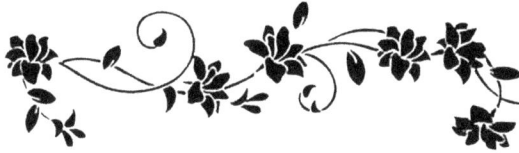

TRAVELING IN MY MIND

I listen to the Dulcimer, Fiddle, and the band
playing the "Westfalia Waltz."
I can see the ladies with their full skirts,
and the men in their starched white shirts,
dancing hand in hand o'er the ballroom floor.
As I listen to the "Mississippi Sawyer,"
I can see dancers clicking their heels
with bodies in motion showing how they feel.
As I hear the "Shepherd's Wife's Waltz,"
I see a young wife, with long shining hair, and skin so fair.
She dances barefoot to the music
that she hears from the breeze
flowing softly through the trees.
The "Flowers of Edinburgh" reminds me
of the Heather as it sways to the music
of the cold wind blowing through
the craigs of the Moorland.
I can travel wherever I choose in my mind,
and it doesn't cost me a dime,
as I listen to the Dulcimer, Fiddle, and the band.

10/22/96

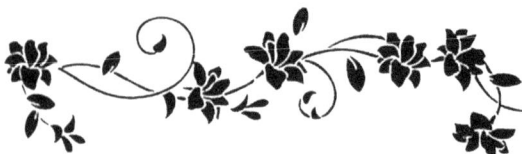

RUNNING AWAY FROM PAIN

There are times that I wish I had wings
So I could fly-fly away up high into the sky
Far away where there'll be no more hurt
Then I realize that's not the answer
For I can't run away from the pain
And loneliness that is embedded inside
Each day I have to begin afresh again
And hide the tears that fall within
I will face the world with a prayer and a smile
And continue to hide the pain that I feel inside

10/29/96

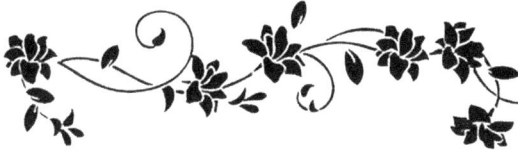

HARVEST TIME

Bails of hay are strewn about the
fields in a beautiful display.
Pumpkins are in the fields nearby
waiting to be chosen for a delicious pie.
The leaves on the trees are turning brown,
and beginning their descent to the waiting ground.
The grass is beginning to die
stating that another year is almost nigh.
Here and there we see rows of corn ready for the harvest.
There are signs of autumn everywhere you look,
with creatures looking for a safe, warm nook.
For some these are signs of sadness,
but we each can look forward to spring with gladness.

10/31/96

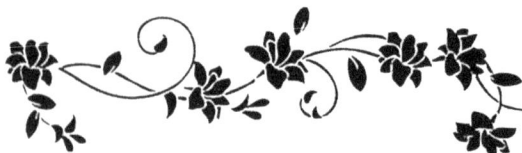

HELP ME PLEASE

As I reached up, You reached down.
I felt the peace and serenity
that can only be found
in the solitude of your Almighty love.
Your arms aren't too short to reach me,
even when I'm down on my knees.
Many times I have to ask you again;
Oh, help me, please!
It seems when I'm at my lowest,
and can't see the light
at the end of the tunnel,
I hear Your voice softly say,
"There's nothing that I can't handle."

12/01/96

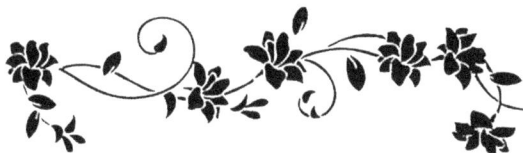

OPEN HEART SURGERY

My heart may be breaking inside,
but there are so many ways that the hurt can be camouflaged.
I wonder if there are different sections of my heart
where each feeling must lodge.
If someone did a triple or quadruple by-pass
of my feelings, which ones would be displayed?
Would it be the insecure feeling
that so many people have;
or would it be the ability to savor each moment;
would it be enjoying the breeze as
it flows through the strands of my hair,
or smelling the fragrance of a rose,
that is floating through the air.
If someone did a triple or quadruple by-pass of my feelings
I would want more happiness than sadness to be found in my heart.

01/16/97

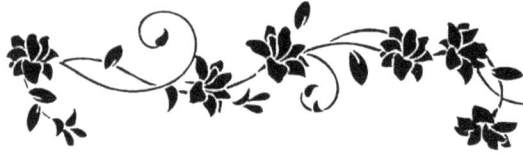

PLEASURES OF A CHILD

Jumping and skipping in the breeze
watching the leaves as they fall from the trees.
Life is like a jungle book
full of changes every where we look.
Sometimes people are like monkeys
who swing from limb to limb,
seeking pleasures that have no end.
Oh, but to be a child again splashing in mud puddles.
Who cares if it gets on our clothes?
It's so much more fun
when we can play in the dirt, and pay no heed.
A child laughs contentedly while following a caterpillar
to see where its' tracks will lead.
There's a part of us that will always remain a child

01/22/97

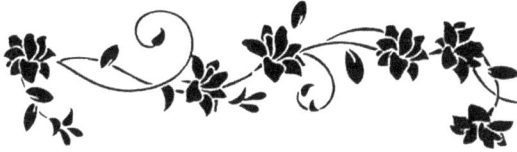

INNERSELF

When you hurt so deeply that it seems no one cares;
If you can find the strength to reach out to someone,
the healing process will begin.
Even while searching for the words to speak,
feelings still inside you keep.
As the thought finally surfaces
and as the tears begin to escape,
a time of purging and renewal
for the soul will evolve.
Even as a segment of your inner self dies,
another segment will branch out into
a new world of its' own.

01/31/97

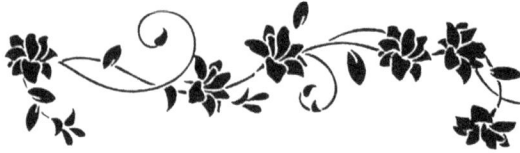

UNDERSTANDING OUR HEART

How well do we know our heart?
It will break in two and we haven't a clue,
as to why it can fall apart
when hit by a love dart.
It can break into pieces without any logical reason.
It's ripe for love during all of the seasons.
It often opens its' door and then wonders what for?
The heart is sometimes used, and often abused.
It should be handled with care and not thrown away,
So it will be there for another day.

02/01/97

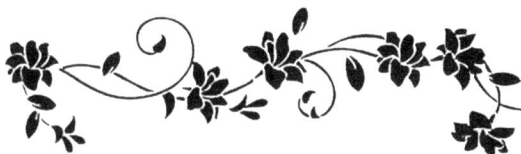

WHAT WAS MAMA THINKING?

I wonder what was on her mind as so long ago
she wrote the words;
"When you see the rainbow at midnight,
and again in the morning,
now is the time to take warning."
Was she remembering things from way back
when that caused her to shed a tear?
"When the birds sing after dark
you had better listen quietly.
You will hear something you don't like."
It isn't unusual to hear birds singing early
in the morning,
but when you hear a dove singing at night,
it sounds so mournful.
"May I in your memory linger like a
sunbeam on the waves.
May I be a friend of yours
'til we meet beyond the grave."
"When this you see please think of me
for in this world I may not be."
She knew her time left on earth was drawing near
as she wrote the thoughts that
I now hold so dear.

02/12/97

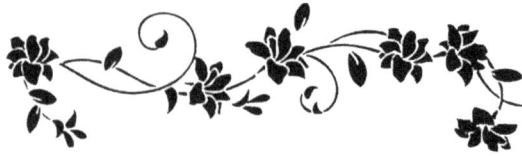

PLANTS AND PEOPLE

People need to be nurtured
just as we care for plants.
We water a plant while it is still green,
as we look forward to the flower
that will eventually appear.
A person needs to be fed daily with love.
The plant without the necessary food and water
will slowly die,
and the flower will never develop.

02/20/97

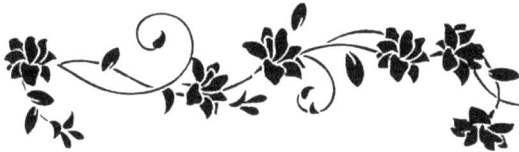

BITTER OR SWEET

The taste of love may be bitter
or it may be sweet.
Either way love is
what makes the heartbeat.
Sometimes it will make you
feel as if you've been hit with an earthquake,
and other times to do a double-take.
Sometimes it will knock you down
and turn you completely around.
It overwhelms you so that you can't utter a sound,
as it tears you apart,
and then puts you back on your feet.
Love can be bitter
or, it can be sweet.

02/24/97

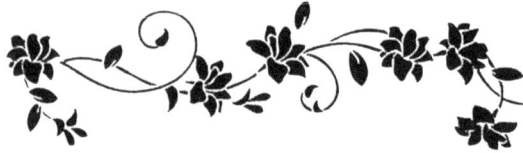

NOWHERE BY ACCIDENT

You go nowhere by accident, so often we've heard,
It just may take you longer to get there.
Certain goals are set in life,
and then you are sidetracked by trouble and strife.
What may seem as the lowest ebb in the tide,
could be the highest wave in the sea.
This wave will carry dreams to shore,
where you attain your goal and so much more.
When it seems all is lost,
and your last dime has been spent,
remember, you go nowhere by accident.

05/04/97

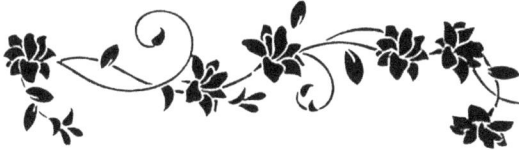

OCEAN WAVES

Ocean waves slowly sing me to sleep,
even as the tentacles pull me into the deep.
Ocean waves around me roll as I struggle to take control.
The sand crystals go wherever they may,
as all the walls I've built around me begin to drift away.
Why fight the octopus anymore,
as the ocean waves around me roar,
And slowly covers me o'er.

07/25/97

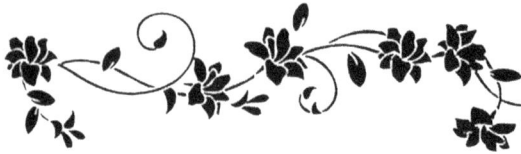

I CAN, I CAN

He sat on the edge of the pool;
could be four or even five.
I think I can, I think I can.
No, I can't, no, I can't.
Thoughts gather in his mind,
As his feet kept rhythm
with the eager hands.
Brother can do this, why can't I?
If he can do it, so can I.
If he can do it, I have to try.
No, I can't, no I can't.
Grandfather with a smile on his face
held out his hand.
I can trust him, I can trust him;
I know I can, I know I can,
as he jumps into the pool.

07/25/97

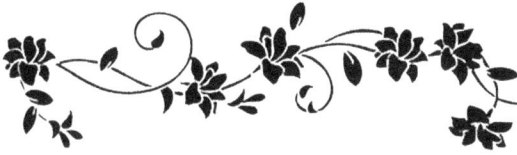

I NEED TO REMEMBER

There are so many times in my life
that I have to step back, Lord,
and let You take control.
After all, you are the One
Who gave your life in ransom for my soul.
In the hustle and bustle of everyday living,
I need to remember who gave me life eternal.

08/15/97

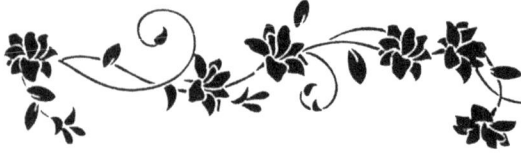

AN OLD SWING

An old swing with tattered rope
hanging from a tree limb
is a reminder of long ago
when laughter of children
could be heard as they swung too and fro.
The old house has been torn down,
and not much sign of a home can be found.
Butterflies and bees are checking
out the roses that were cared for
so lovingly, that now are
left behind.
An old swing, a tattered rope, a rose;
another place,
another time.

08/22/97

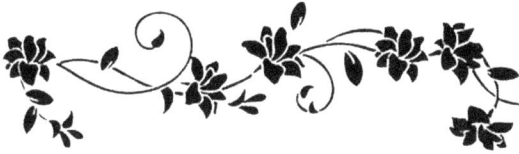

ANOTHER DAY

The sun is playing peek a boo
with me this morning
as it slowly awakens me with its'
fingers softly stroking my eyelashes.
Even as I snuggle beneath the covers
for just one more minute,
the bright rays gently caress
my body with its' warmth.
I can no longer lie idle.
I have been given another day
to rise and make of it
whatever I may.

09/12/97

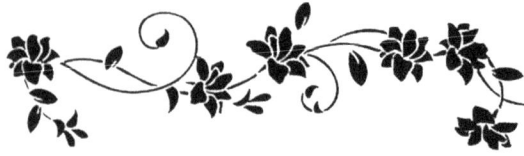

BRUISED FAMILY

Last year she held her side when she coughed;
Must have been the way she lay in her bed.
A few months ago, she brought a new baby
home from the hospital.
Oh, please, not tonight!
Last month she had a black eye,
and bruises on her face;
She fell down the steps.
Last week she had a black eye, bruises,
And a cut on her leg.
Little boy or little girl doesn't seem
to fit in at school;
Notes sent home to parents.
What's wrong with you?
Why don't you make good grades?
Can't you do anything right?
Little boy goes to school limping;
Little girl goes to school with black eye.

09/15/97

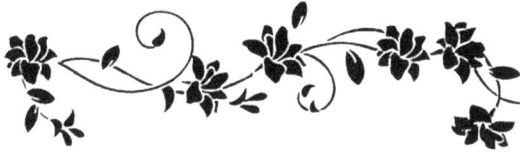

THE BATTERED SHIP

Her body has been battered and torn
by life's sharks
She has been a ship bearing the love of God.
Slaves of sin have been
set free from the shackles that bound them.
The captain of the ship is the
Master of the sea,
and can calm the raging storms
and waves that threaten to sink.
When the time comes to tow
the ship into harbor,
the Anchor will hold, and
the Helmsman will guide her
safely into the shore.

09/16/97

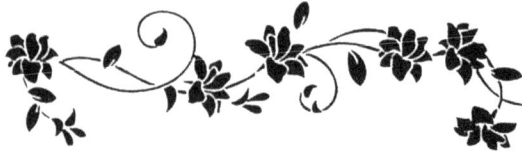

SURVIVAL

Sometimes circumstances seemed to be
out of control,
and to deal with it would take
some one very bold.
When the time for decisions
came to sink, swim, or die,
I did what I had to do
in order to survive—
and then I wondered why.

09/22/97

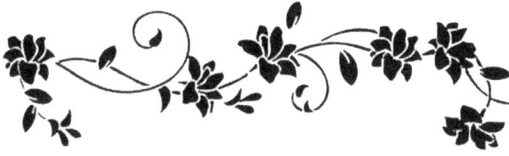

I'LL NEVER WALK ALONE

I felt the need to be alone,
so I went for a walk where I once called home.
As I wondered aimlessly letting my thoughts meander,
scenes from my childhood, I began to remember.
I traveled the path that I walked as a child,
and those times I now recall with a smile.
The daisies are blooming, and the fragrance of
Honeysuckles fill the air.
Those were the days when I didn't have a care.
The music of the Robin floats along with the breeze
as I try to find them among the trees.
My footsteps find their way to the creek
where the cool water flows o'er my feet.
Much to my surprise and delight, a shikepoke
is startled out of its reverie and immediately takes flight.
When I feel the need to be alone,
I go for a walk where I once called home,
only to realize, Lord with You by my side,
I'll never need to walk alone.

12/04/97

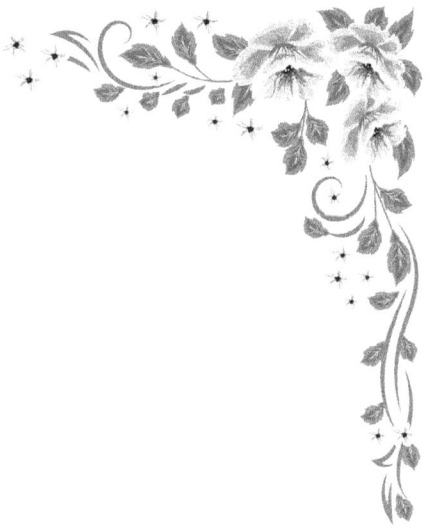

MODERATE - SEVERE STAGE

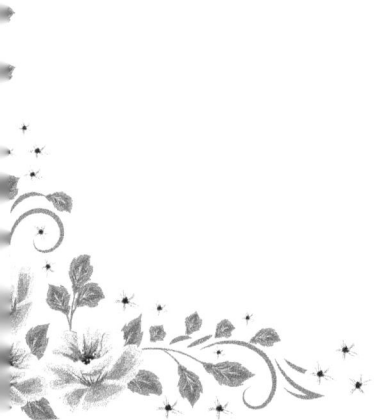

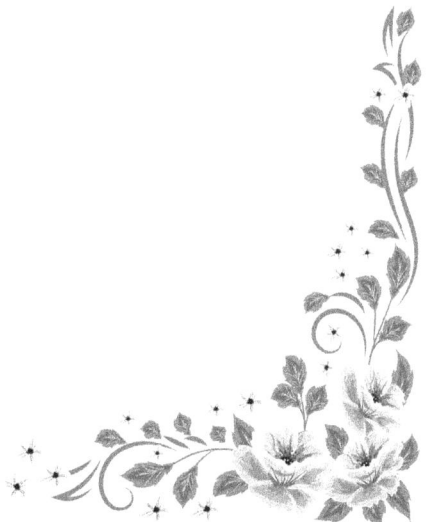

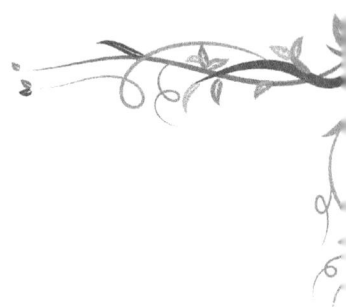

12/18/97

Ken went to the farm to bush hog, and tried to cut some plastic off that was there for a reason. In the process, he jabbed the knife into his wrist. I didn't know until I came home how bad it was. He wouldn't let me call the doctor. He had gone to the drugstore, and the pharmacist told him to put an antibiotic on it, and thought it would be alright.

12/19/97

I called the doctor, and they saw Ken today. He was sent to Dr. McGowan who wanted an opinion on possible nerve damage, as Ken had no feeling in the lower half of his hand.

12/20/97

Ken kept rubbing his hand and saying it feels numb.

12/21/97

Ken kept rubbing his hand and hasn't slept well the last two nights.

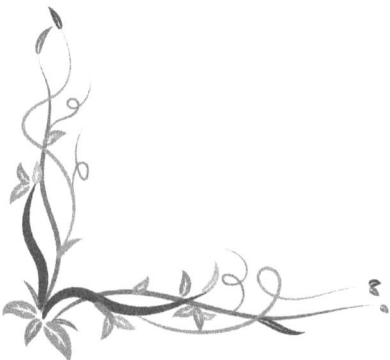

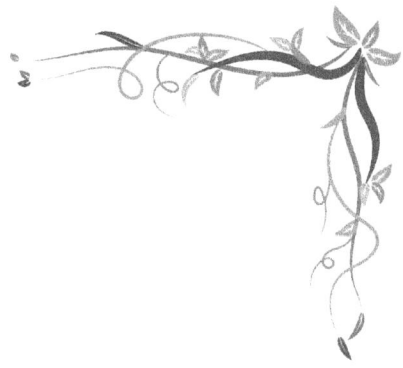

12/22/97

Ken went to King to have work done on his truck. I told him if it was over $200.00 to call me before he wrote a check. When he came in later, he had written the check for almost $600.00. I panicked. I called, and asked them to hold until the next day, so I could get the money out of savings.

In the meantime, Dr. McGowan's office called to say we had an appointment today to see Dr. Pollock, and that it was extremely important that we kept it. He said that Ken needed surgery which was scheduled for 12/29/97.

After we came home, Ken constantly asked for the date of his surgery. Tomorrow he goes for pre-op registration. He keeps wanting to know where he is supposed to go, and then doesn't remember where Medical Park is located. Finally, out of the clear blue, he said, "Why didn't you tell me it's between Forsyth Hospital, and where I had my sinus surgery?"

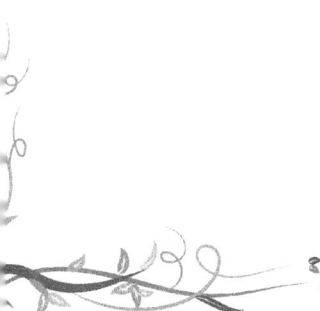

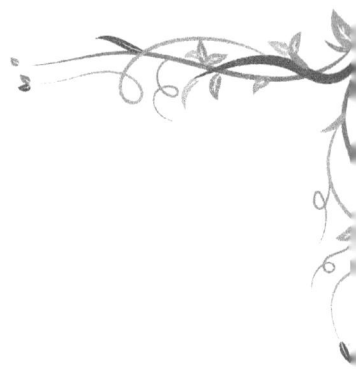

12/23/97

The morning of Ken's lab work, I drove so I could go on to work. He was waiting for me, and said, "They're not going to do my surgery today." He just couldn't understand why not. I tried to explain to him again. All that week he kept asking what day is my surgery, what time, etc. He also couldn't remember where Medical Park was located. He did fine with his surgery. He had vacation to take before the end of the year.

My friend, Donna was determined that I'd have a gift from Ken this Christmas, so she talked with him at length one night on the phone about what he could get me. She told me later that he asked her to check on the price, which she did. She then called to tell him. They talked a long time, and I could tell he was becoming very frustrated.

Ken finally handed me the phone. She said, "Polly, Ken is confused. Don't say anything." She then asked me to try to talk to him, because he thought that I already had the Pilot Mountain earrings. He had given me the Pilot Mountain necklace. I talked with him and told him three things that I thought she may be talking about, and that I had mentioned to her that I would like to have the Pilot Mountain earrings. He said, "Oh, let me call her back, I know now what to tell her." He called her, and she later told me that he seemed alright.

I told Donna when Ken paid her, if it wasn't enough to let me know, and I would pay the rest. She wrapped the earrings in a small box, and had also bought a jacket, which she wrapped. He picked them up at her house, but didn't remember what was in the gifts, or who they were for. He also couldn't remember how they got under our Christmas tree. This is so frustrating for both of us.

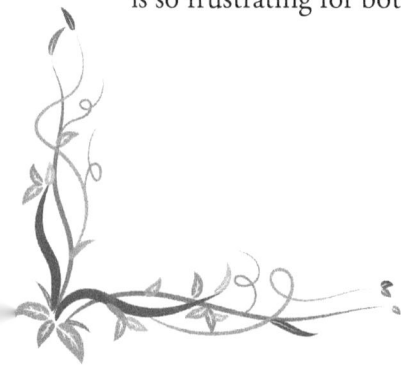

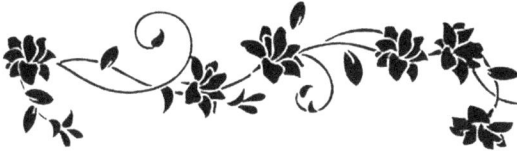

SMILE OF A CHILD

The sweet smile of a child makes life worthwhile.
At the end of a long weary day as the door closes behind you
a little voice says,
"Please come and play with me."
There are so many reasons why you just can't,
but so many reasons why you can.
You can't relive today,
and tomorrow your child may not want to play.
Take advantage of the blessings you have today,
for they could easily be taken away.

12/26/97

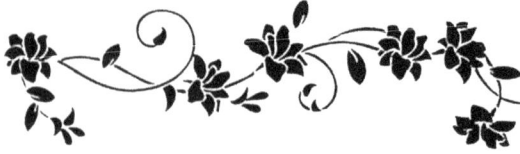

THE OLD HOMEPLACE

The old home place is not as it was
when we as kids played with our handmade toys.
Brother with a broken broom stick
that he rode for a horse, and
I with my corn shuck doll would be playing nearby.
The land is all grown up where we once planted corn,
and some people would not know that this was
once a thriving farm.
The old feed barn is falling down where the hay
in the hayloft was cozy as down.
The Chevy truck all rusty and worn,
is parked in the Honeysuckles snug and warm.
It's a reminder of times shared when we as kids
felt safe from harm.

01/01/98

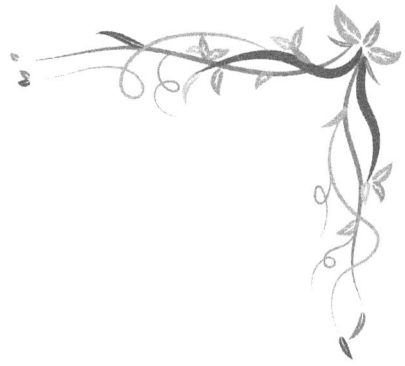

01/01/98

Our water pump was cutting on and off, so I asked Ken who I needed to call. He said "There's nothing wrong with it. Finally, after lunch he let me call our friend who worked on it for a long time, and thought he had it fixed. This is so difficult.

01/02/98

The pump still is not working right, but Ken won't let me tell anyone. We went shopping with Kenny and Donna. Ken did pretty well.

01/03/98

The water pump is really messed up. Ken did let me call Kenny again after lunch. He didn't want me to call anyone else. Kenny worked on it until 9:00 P.M., and it still is not right. Kenny and I both called a plumber, but neither returned our call.

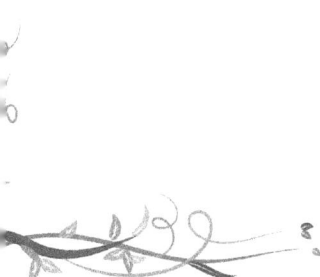

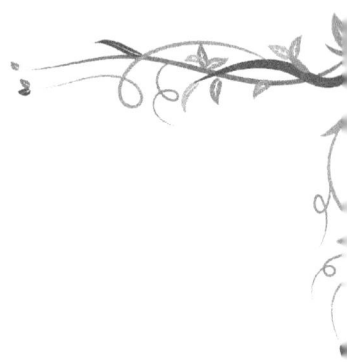

01/05/98

When I came in from work, I asked Ken if anyone came today. He said, "No, and nobody called." I called the plumber again, and left a message. Ken then said, "I know what's wrong with the pump." I asked, "What?" He said, "The generator is messed up." I asked him "How do you know?" He said, "That's what the man said today," and looked at me as if he knew what he was talking about. I asked, "What man?" He said, "It must have been Kenny's friend, I don't know his name. He goes to Friendly Chapel." I asked, "Is he coming tomorrow to fix it?" He looked real confused, and said, "I don't know."

01/06/98 -

I called the plumber, and he said, "Didn't your husband tell you that I came yesterday?" I explained Ken's memory problems, and he apologized. He said, "He acted as if he knew me the first time I came, but the second time he acted as if he had no idea who I was, nor why I was there."

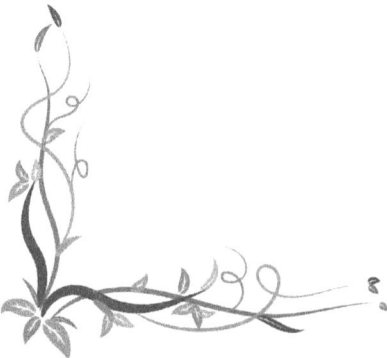

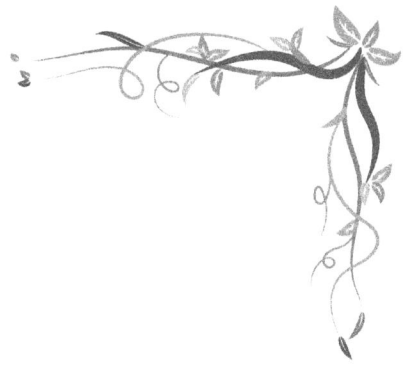

01/09/98

Ken kept asking if I had gotten a bill from the plumber. When I came home today, he was sitting in his chair staring at the T.V. I asked if he wanted to go out to eat with Kenny and Donna. He said, "I don't know. Did you get a bill from the plumber?" I said, "Yes, I paid it today." He asked, "How much did he charge?" When I told him, he said, "I didn't want you to pay him, because he took $35.00 worth of my pipe." I tried to reason with him, and get him calmed down. I finally said, "I'll call Donna and tell her that we won't eat with them." He said, "Why not?" I said, "If you're going to act like this, I don't want to go." He said, "We'll go." He was withdrawn all evening. He usually enjoys playing Rook with Donna and Kenny, but it is becoming difficult to follow him.

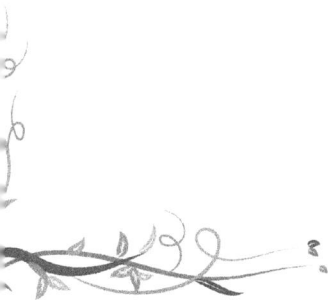

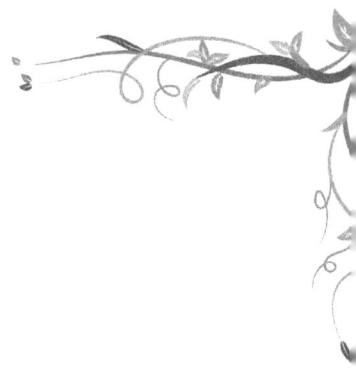

01/10/98

I went to rent a video, and saw one of the men who works with Ken. He asked about him, as he is still out of work from his wrist surgery. I asked Tom how Ken did at work, and tears came into his eyes. He said "Some days he was as he had always been, and other days, he just couldn't get it together. He would become real frustrated. Some of the men who have known him for years watch for the signs, and will talk to him to get him calmed down. Four of the men, who drive to work from Mount Airy, and from Pilot Mountain, watch for him each morning to make sure he gets to work."

01/11/98

We didn't go to Sunday School this morning, but went to worship service. Angel and the quartet wanted to meet at the church and practice at 5:00 P.M. I went to walk for one hour, came home to check on Ken, and then went to church. He doesn't always want to go with me when we practice. I came home about 7:00 P.M. Ken wouldn't speak when I walked in, and appeared to be pouting with me. I ignored him for a while, and gradually tried to draw him out of it. Eventually he seemed alright.

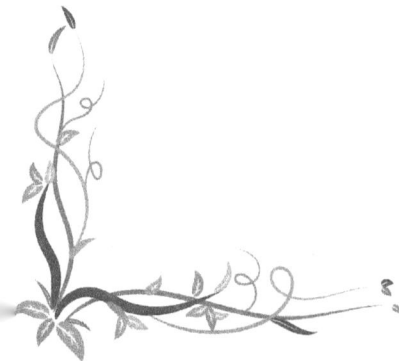

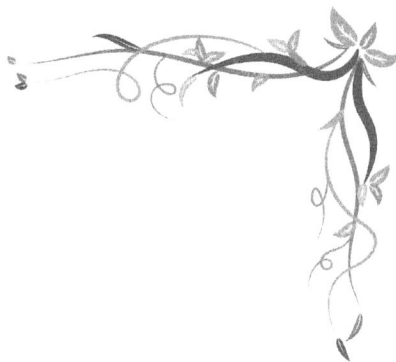

01/22/98

Ken was so angry with me tonight. He originally had an appointment today for a second opinion with Dr. Creeger. Since he had already had surgery, Dr. Creeger's office said there was no need to come.

Ken's hand is still really red and tender, and he still doesn't have feeling in his little finger. He accused me of telling the doctor that he didn't need to see him, and that I cancelled his appointment. He was taking his frustration out on me. I finally just walked out of the room, as there is no need to argue with him.

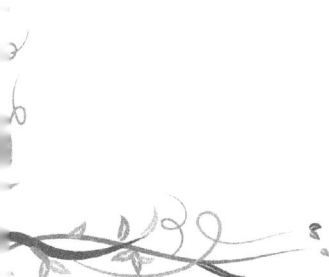

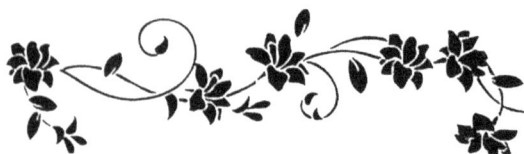

EMPTY SPACE IN HEAVEN

There must have been a large empty space in Heaven
when Jesus came to earth.
He filled a special place among men,
then one day He gave His life in order to save them.
Sometimes we get a glimpse of the
S-U-N behind a cloud that reminds me
of the S-O-N Who left behind an empty
tomb, and a discarded shroud.
How the angels must have rejoiced
when His work on earth was completed,
and He returned home leaving the Holy Spirit to comfort us,
so we'd never be alone.

01/23/98

****

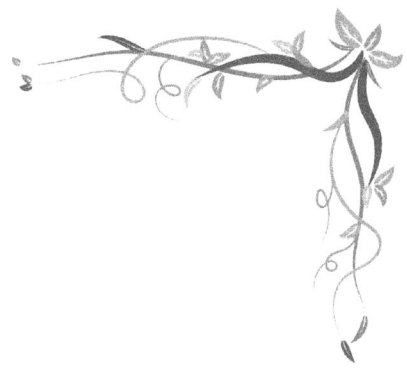

01/24/98

We went to Donna and Kenny's. When we arrived, Ken kept looking for the car door handle. He looked around at me, and said, "Don't you laugh." If he only knew, how badly I wanted to cry.

01/25/98

Ken sang in the church choir this morning, but I noticed he kept looking for me. It seemed when he could see me, he would relax.

01/26/98

Ken went back to work this morning. He seemed nervous. I'm uneasy about him, but I am limited.

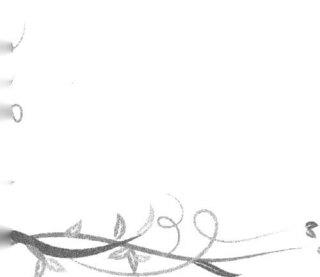

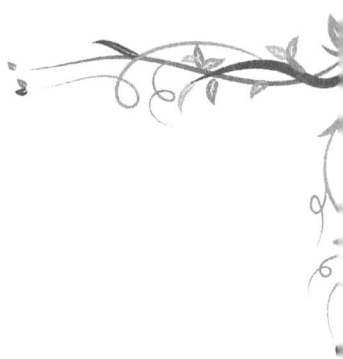

03/01/98

I was coming out of our bathroom, and Ken started dancing around with his fists swinging toward me, and said, "Do you wanna fight?" I said "No, but I think you do." He said, "Honey, I wouldn't hurt you, I love you too much."

These mood swings are not easy to deal with. Ken's truck has been out of commission for about four weeks now. He questions every move I make. He wants to know where I'm going, and when I'm coming home.

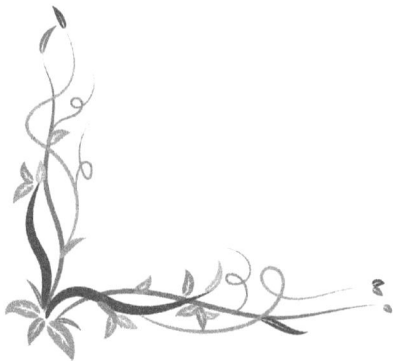

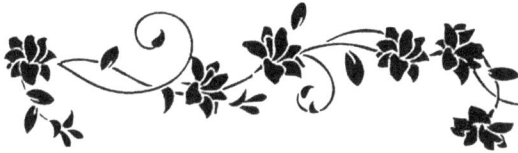

WHAT I LEAVE BEHIND

When on earth I fall asleep to wake no more,
I'll awake to live forever on God's golden shore.
Many times the sea of life has been so rough
I could hardly hang on,
but, then I'd see the light from the Lighthouse
and I knew I wasn't alone.
No matter how high the waves may toss,
my soul is anchored to the cross.
All will not be lost when my life is o'er,
if what I leave behind
leads someone to Heaven forever more.

03/10/98

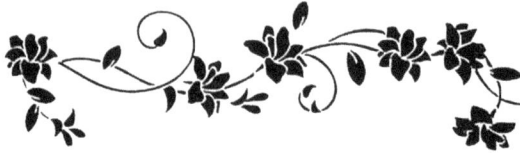

PEBBLE ON THE BEACH

If I could be anything other than whom I am,
I think I'd like to be a pebble on the beach
where I could bask in the warm sunshine
and let the grains of sand and water flow o'er me.
With no concept of time
I would be in the fresh air,
and wouldn't have a care.
I would be close to nature, and
could reach out and touch the sea creatures.
I could drift with the tide as the
warm sea breeze softly caressed me.
Oft times I wish I could be
A pebble on the beach, but
I suppose it's best that we can't choose
who or what we are to be.

03/13/98

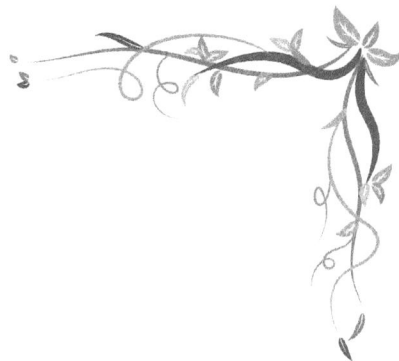

03/14/98

I drove Ken to Dad's for them to go to Mount Airy. Ken questioned me several times as to where I was going. I kept telling him to get my nails done, and that I'd be home about 2:00 P.M. When I came home about 1:00 P.M., he would hardly speak to me. Donna had called, and wanted me to go shopping with her. I told Ken that we'd be gone until about 5:00 P.M., and asked if he wanted me to leave him a note. He was rather abrupt with his answer of No! I had also told him if he wanted to watch the ball game with Kenny to go on down there.

Donna called Kenny to meet us at Pizza Hut at 6:00 P.M. When they met us, Ken wouldn't speak to me. I could tell he was upset. As soon as we were in the car to go home, he turned to me, and said. "OK., I want to know where you have been, and what you have been doing. You've been gone all day." I reminded him that I had offered to leave a note for him, and that I didn't want to hear any more about it. He then began talking as if nothing had happened.

03/15/98

Ken went to church today, and has been rather quiet. I told him that he had an appointment with the dentist Wednesday at 1:30 P.M. I wrote a note and put it on the table.

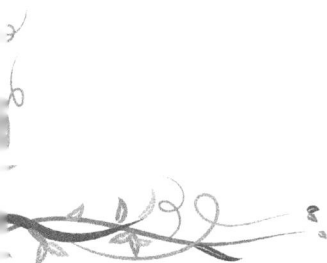

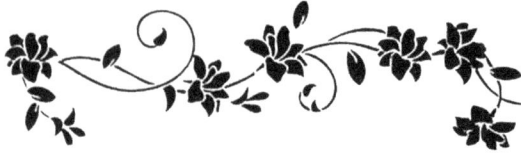

LU CHEN

She reminded me of a butterfly
as she zoomed from side to side
with arms flung open wide
when she would glide so gracefully
across the ice with such a serene
look upon her face.
No one but those close to her would
know what it had cost this
young girl to come back all these miles
for the last two years.
With the good luck charm around her neck
from her boyfriend,
this young girl named Lu Chen
fulfilled a dream against all odds,
and arrived back home with the Bronze.

03/17/98

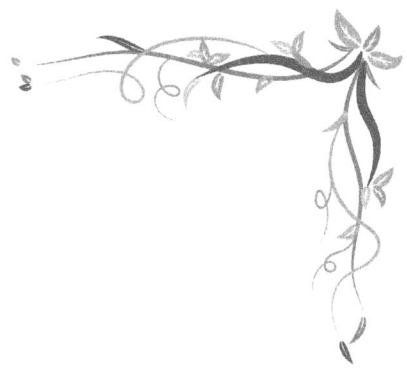

03/17/98

I left a note for Ken this morning to find when he came home from work. I told him that I would be late tonight as I was getting my hair cut. When I walked in the door, he jumped up out of his chair and said, "The next time you make an appointment, make it after I get off work." I tried to explain to him that we can't always do that. Then he said, "And the next time, don't wait until the last minute to tell me. I called and cancelled." He then went out the door. He came back in and I said, "I wait to tell you so you won't be worrying about it, and then forget." He said, "If I forget, it's my problem." He forgot his coat, and when he came back in to get it, he was so upset he was shaking. I didn't say any more to him. I ate, took my bath and went to bed. I know how frustrating this is for me, and it has to be worse for him.

03/18/98

This morning as Ken went out the door to work, he said, "You need to call, and cancel my appointment. I reminded him that he told me last night that he had called and cancelled. An odd look came over his face, and he said, "Well, maybe I did."

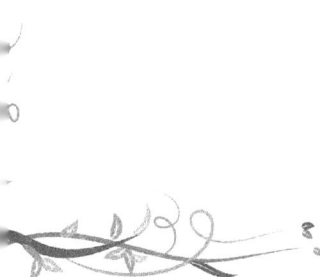

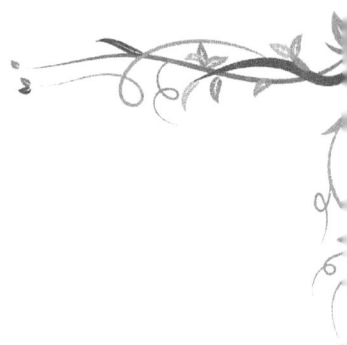

03/27/98

My friend, Donna, was going on a trip to the beach for a prayer retreat with other women from her church. There was a cancellation at the last minute, and she asked me to go. It was a blessing in disguise. (Her husband and Ken were going to spend time together, so Ken wouldn't be alone.) We spent time in prayer, studying our Bibles, listening to special singing, and encouragement from speakers. I wrote this next poem as we were traveling.

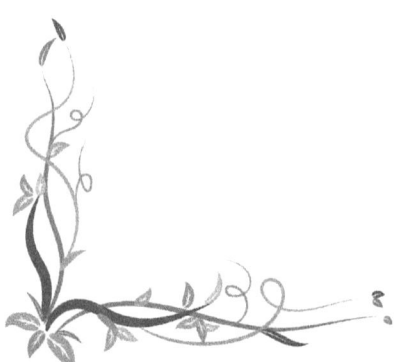

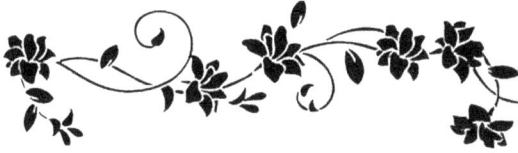

ON A MISSION

Donna, Margaret, Barbara, and I
set out on a mission like steadfast troubadours.
We filled the trunk with suitcases full of clothes,
and more clothes.
Of course, a mission is not complete
without lots of good food to eat.
There's bathroom time, break time,
and all around fun time.
As we traveled and viewed the handiwork of God,
we were in awe with the beauty that He provides.
We shared anecdotes of happy times, and
touched briefly on sad.
We looked for road signs to make sure
we were on the right track.
We wanted to be equipped to find our way back.
Our road of life is oft times filled with curves, and dips,
but when we follow God's road map,
we are fully equipped.

03/27/98

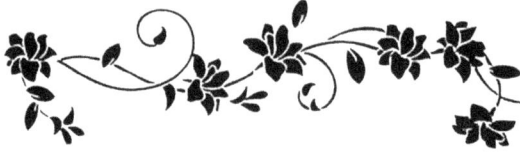

LIFE IS NOT ALWAYS FAIR

My world is slowly tearing apart.
My heart is being ripped open.
The sphere around me seems
as cold as the breeze from the ocean waves
on a dark March night.
The frothy white bubbles
are slowly pulling at the sand
and separating the particles wherever it can.
I shiver in the chilled night air,
as my heart cries out,
Life is not always fair.

03/27/98

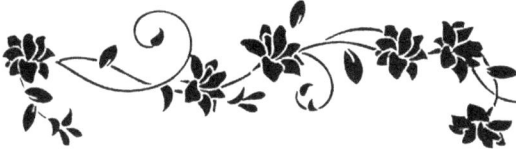

IN THE EYE OF THE STORM

When we're in the eye of the storm,
Jesus is calm.
When we don't know which way to turn,
Jesus is right.
When our life is full of turmoil,
Jesus is peace.
When part of the puzzle is missing,
Jesus can put it together.
Lord, we give to you
All praise and glory!

03/28/98

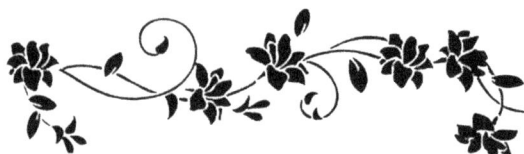

WHERE OTHERS FEAR TO TREAD

Jesus was an earthly carpenter's son
Who came to earth to see
that His Heavenly Father's work was done.
He brought with him all of the necessary tools.
He had a forgiving heart,
and was willing to do His part.
His feet walked where others feared to tread,
as they found their way to the cross,
where there His blood was shed.
He arose from the borrowed tomb,
and returned to His Heavenly throne.
There He would wait until
His beloved ones were called home.

04/08/98

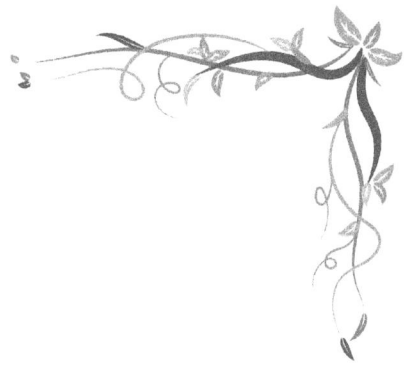

07/05/98

Ken woke me up during the night brushing off the foot of the bed on my side. He kept mumbling something, and when I spoke to him, he lay back down, but he tossed and turned all night.

07/14/98

Ken's dental hygienist at Dr. Clark's office called to tell me that the new secretary had called Ken at work to remind him of his appointment on Thursday, the 16th. About one-half hour later, she called to tell me that he had just come, and thought it was today. A short time later, he came to where I work with a puzzled expression. He doesn't like to miss work, so I told him to go on back, as he would have to be off Thursday.

07/16/98

I wrote Ken a note to put in his pocket to remind him of his appointment today. He came home this afternoon, and said he had to leave his upper plate at Dr. Clark's office in the morning at 7:00 A.M. He had asked to be off work tomorrow. I kept questioning him about the time, and date, and did he have a card. He kept saying, no. About one-half hour later, he pulled a card out of his billfold, and his appointment is Monday, July 20th.

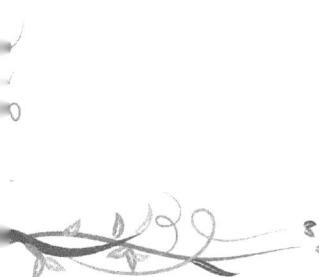

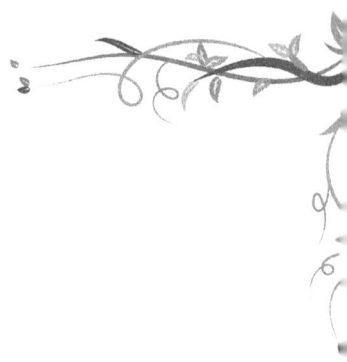

07/17/98

Ken went to work today. As we were eating supper, I asked him if he remembered to ask off for Monday, and he couldn't remember.

07/25/98

Ken played golf with Kenny today. Donna later told me that Kenny told her that Ken kept trying to take the flagpole to the golf cart. Kenny is noticing Ken's increasing confusion.

07/26/98

When I went into our Sunday School class this morning, Ken had already sat down. As I began to sit down beside him, he jerked the chair, and threw me off balance. He laughed and said, "But you still love me, don't you?" He thought it was funny, but I didn't.

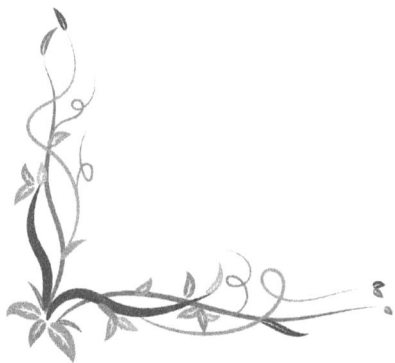

09/98

Ken has been seen by Dr. Roach, his medical doctor, Dr. Crowell, Neurology Specialist, Dr. Weaver, Psychiatrist, and Dr. Pepper, Psychologist, at different intervals. Each did their own evaluation, ruling out certain medical problems, and prescribed medication accordingly. We both were so weary from going for test after test. Dr. Pepper was asked to do a Neuropsychological Evaluation in September 1998. The results showed Ken had generalized and severe memory impairment, decline in intellectual abilities, and generalized attentional impairment. The results were judged to be consistent with a neuro-degenerative process such as Alzheimer's disease.

(The Alzheimer's Association sent me the book "The 36 Hour Day," which should be very helpful.)

My mammogram was scheduled for October 08, 1998. I arrived at my scheduled time, chatted with employees, and made small talk with other women who were waiting to be "compressed."

One lady was concerned when she was asked to have another test. I tried to console her by telling her that each year I had extra pictures taken. When my name was called, I was fine, and then, I had to have another, and then another. By this time, I wasn't so brave. The other lady was fine, for which I was thankful. The doctor showed me the x-ray that told him something, and by this time, I was definitely nervous. A biopsy was scheduled for Thursday.

A call came from Dr. Pennell on October 13, 1998, stating, "You have localized metastasis cancer in the milk gland. We found it in time and it is treatable." Of course, all I heard was the big "C" word. At first, denial, then questions with no answers. What will become of me? Will I need a mastectomy or lumpectomy? When I arrived home, I headed to my special meditation place, and there I was reassured that God would be with me. Fortunately, my oncologist Dr. Ferree, was very understanding as we reviewed the options, and settled for the lumpectomy, unless there were complications.

What is this enemy
that has invaded my body?
Will it be here only temporarily,
or has it come to stay for a party?
Tears turned to rivers
My whole being shivers
Partly from pain
Partly from fear
What will happen to this form
that my Mom once held so near?

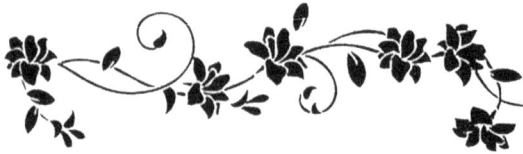

OLD FAMILIAR FACES

My thoughts and my heart draw
me back to the old home place.
As I wondered aimlessly drawing
strength from the quietness,
there was something missing.
Where are the old familiar faces,
and the sound of their laughter?
Where are the voices calling out to each other?
They are in the deep crevices of my mind
where forever they shall be.
The wildflowers of such beauty
soon wither and are gone,
but the seeds that fall to the earth
will bloom again another year.
So will the memory of you live on.

09/21/98

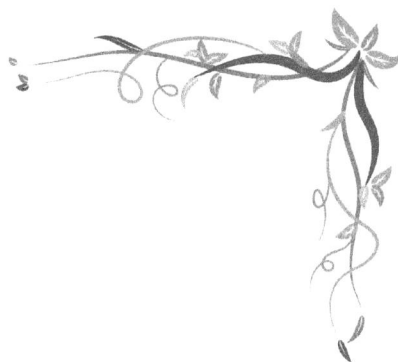

10-14-98

Surgery was scheduled for October 28, 1998. I remember standing in front of the mirror surveying my body for the last time before surgery. I knew in my heart that I was God's creation, and He could mold it as He chose. I just wasn't sure how that would be.

Of course, as any woman would be, I was concerned with who would do the washing of clothes, cleaning the house, cooking, etc. My husband having previously been diagnosed with Alzheimer's, concerned me. Every need was met. Food appeared as if by magic, the house was cleaned as if by elves, and so many necessary things done by such wonderful people. I did have to give instructions to Ken as to where the silverware was located, what to take out of the refrigerator, where the plates were, how much to put on the plates, and what option to push on the microwave. It was difficult, but we survived.

I remember awakening still groggy from the anesthesia, and all I could see was Doctor Pennell's eyes and feel his hand patting mine. He said, "I think we have it all, but we will have to await the lab results." The cancer was two inches in depth, and was so small, that if I hadn't had the mammogram, the cancer would have spread before I would have become aware. The first thing that I did upon awakening in my room was to feel to see if I still had a breast. A dear friend, Darla, who was with me said, "Yes, you still have it."

Even while I was still trying to awaken, the phone rang, and I heard a familiar concerned voice. I drifted back to sleep with a smile.

The surgery is over and scars are healing. I have heard all of my life that an ounce of prevention is worth a pound of cure. When Dr. Pennell told me that all was well, I was reassured that the mammogram was well worth the time.

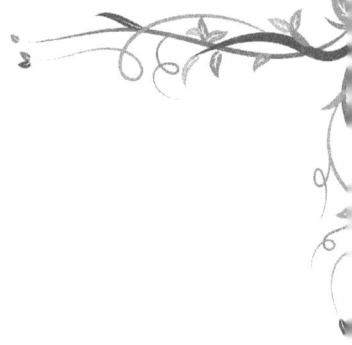

I lie in a somewhat comatose state,
thoughts whirling as they consider my fate.
Sounds floating around me from where, I'm not sure.
Is it too much to ask for a cure?
Familiar voices swirl in and out,
as they talk o'er my sleeping body.
I want to know the prognosis—
but then again, I'm not sure that I'm ready.
The doctor gently pats me on the hand,
and in his kind voice says,
"we think we got it all, but we're not sure yet."
Outwardly the scars are healing,
inwardly my body is reeling.
What is this enemy that has invaded my body?
Has it come to visit temporarily,
or will it stay and have a party?

11-01-98

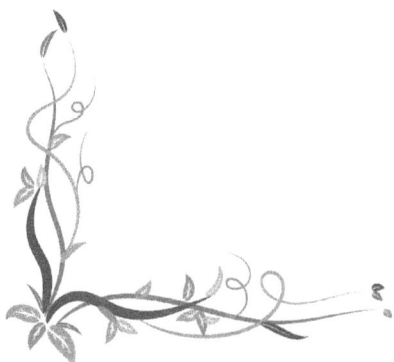

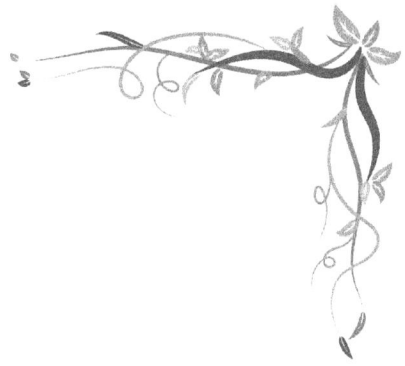

I lie quietly awaiting the
doctor's entrance into the room.
What will be the outcome?
Will they have the results this soon?
Thru my mind so many thoughts
and questions are fighting for attention.
The doctor enters the room in his usual brisk pace,
reading the reports from this his current case.
Was this ounce of prevention worth a pound of cure?
When I hear the answer I respond with
"Are you sure? Are you sure?"
The ounce of prevention was worth the pound of cure.
Women who feel that it's a waste of time
to have their mammogram each year,
only needs to weigh the odds,
and spare their loved ones many tears.

11-04-98

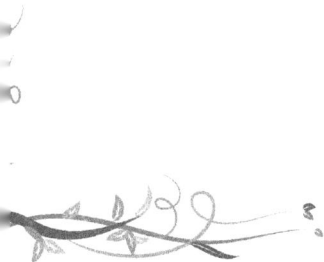

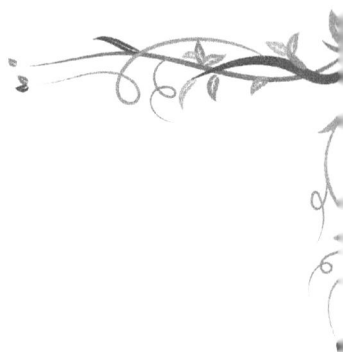

When we're born into this world
we aren't promised a life
without pain or without heartache,
but, when trials do arise
God will be there to provide.

11-10-98

****

I lie gazing at the bright red light
waiting any moment to be escorted
up by the aliens who are
surely hiding in this room.
I keep thinking "Beam me up Scottie,"
as I chuckle and say to myself
I've not been in anyone's toddy."
I lie quietly and don't make a sound
as the planning laser beams make their rounds.
I am told to breathe normally,
but I am not sure anymore
what is normal.

12-07-98

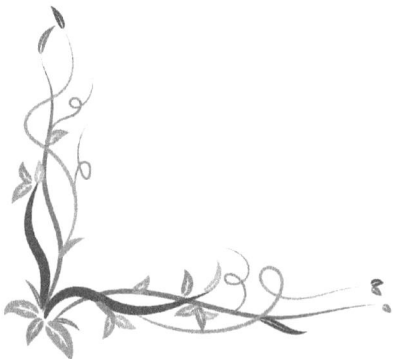

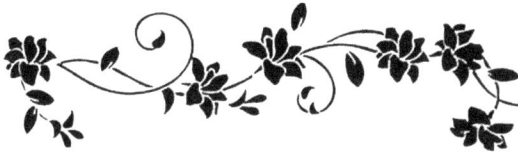

FACE OF A GNOME

An old tree stripped naked
had such a desolate appearance.
Crooked, knarled arms reached
out to nearby trees for assurance.
It appeared to have survived
many stark, cold, lonely winters
with determination.
It must have provided shelter
for numerous generations of
birds and squirrels, as they
built their nests among the branches.
What comfort they must have felt
as they snuggled safe and warm,
embraced by this old tree
that now wears a face of
desolation and looks like a gnome.

11-19-98

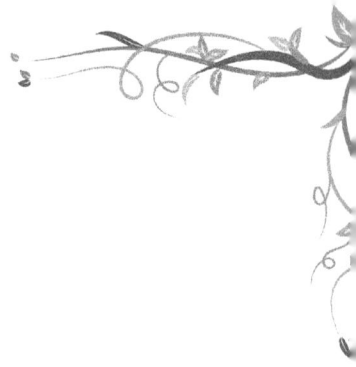

I was most fortunate that I only had to take radiation for six weeks with no chemo.

This morning I am so tired
and all I want to do is sleep.
Reality awakens me
and tells me that I must at least try.
Even as I do, I fight the urge to cry.
So many events are taking place
that is out of my control.

12-22-98

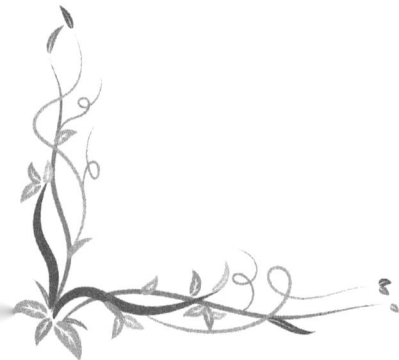

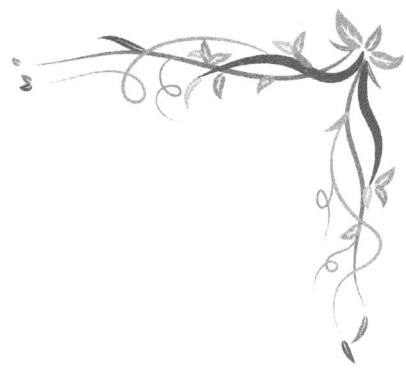

My knees are wobbly
and my body is weak.
It seems that I keep tripping
all o'er my feet.
They're only a size 4,
but at times they feel
like they're two x fours.

01-22-99

****

My body aches
and I keep thinking
how much more can I take!
I do believe my body
is falling apart bit by bit.
Could it be rebuilt
if someone purchased a kit?

01-25-99

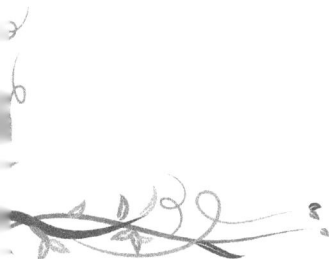

Hurray!!!!!! By the end of January, I am back in the running.

TO MAKE YOUR DREAMS COME TRUE

Dream big!
Dig Deep!
Never give up!!!

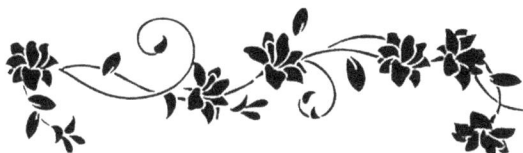

I FEEL SO ALONE

I feel so alone
and my eyes are full of tears.
My heart is breaking inside
as another part of me dies.
I need someone to go home
to at night,
someone who will hold me close,
and make everything alright.
There is no one I can go to, Lord.
Where are you?
I don't feel that you hear me anymore.

03/12/99

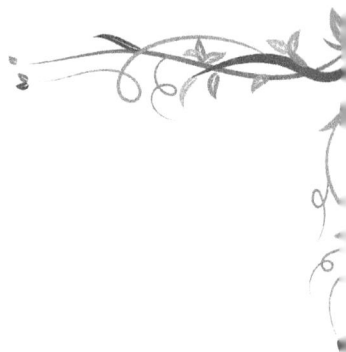

08/18/99

When I came home from work, Ken said "I got in trouble at work today, and Justin told me to stay home tomorrow, cool off, and come back Thursday." When I asked what he'd done, he said "Gary kept aggravating me, and I had to go outside to keep from hurting him." Ken has threatened different times to jab a wrench down his throat, or something similar. He kept asking me after that if he had to go to work tomorrow, and I'd tell him no.

08/19/99

When I came home from work, Ken began asking if he had to go to work tomorrow, and I said, "Yes."

08/20/99

Ken didn't want to go to work today. He was real nervous. When I got home from work, he said, "I told Freddy I'm taking vacation the rest of the week."

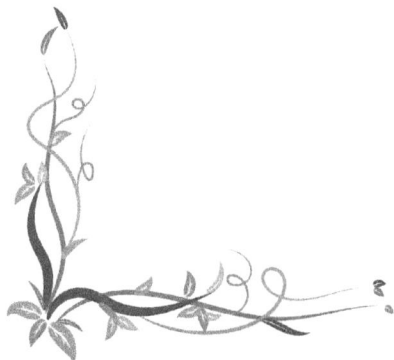

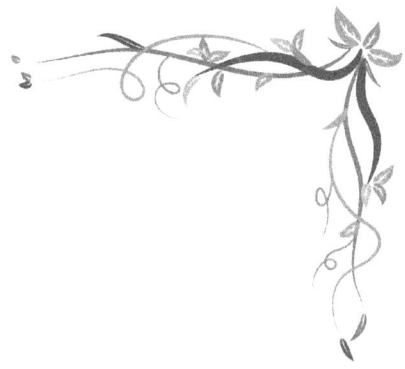

08/24/99

Ken has asked several times this weekend if he has to go to work Monday. I told him I'd call for him. He has vacation he can take. He seemed relieved, and then he'd ask the same question again.

08/25/99

I called Carol at Champion and told her that Ken would take vacation this week. (He never went back to work.) I called Dr. Weaver's office and told his secretary what was happening, and he set Ken up for another evaluation with Dr. Pepper, who did one a year ago. Ken said he didn't want to quit work, but that he doesn't have to worry as much about being confused and getting in trouble.

EPHESIANS 4:30

AND GRIEVE NOT THE HOLY SPIRIT OF GOD, WHEREBY YE ARE SEALED UNTO THE DAY OF REDEMPTION.

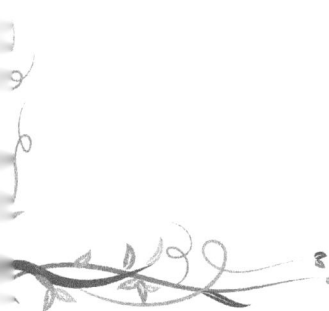

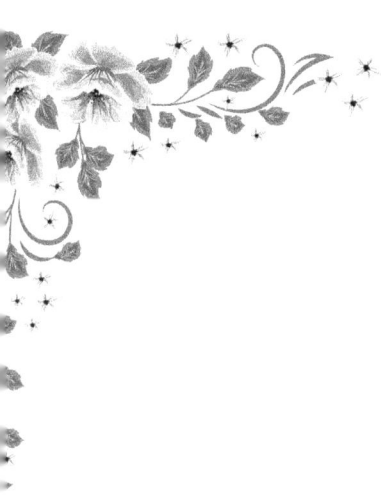

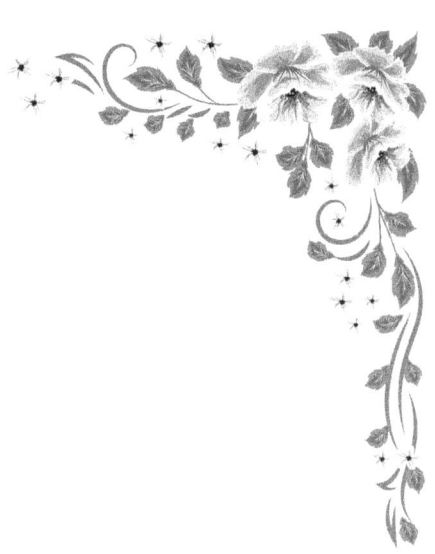

SEVERE – FINAL STAGE

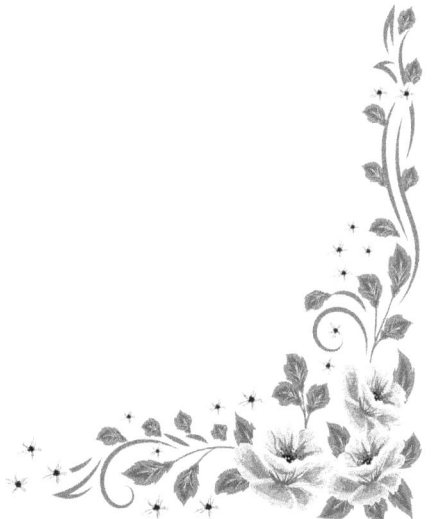

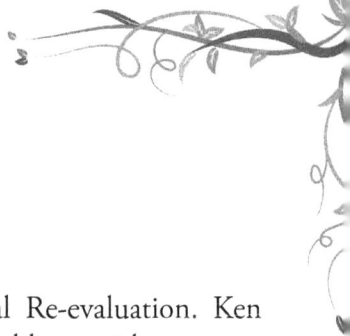

10/22/99

Dr. Pepper did another Neuropsychological Re-evaluation. Ken shared with her that he had a lack of energy, problems with memory, incontinence, word-finding problems, a sense that familiar things are strange or unreal, inability to read, write, spell, or calculate, and feelings of worthlessness. He stated to her "my head's messed up," and admitted that he is having difficulty performing his job. He told her that a co-worker is "messing" with him, such as rearranging his tools or his machine when he is not looking. He also admitted that "I'm gonna kill him the next time he does that." He was cooperative during the testing session, but was easily frustrated.

Dr. Pepper recommended that he be placed in a locked facility for Alzheimer's patients that provided 24-hour supervision. He was declared to be in the late-stage Alzheimer's disease. She said Ken needs to apply for disability, and that she'd send me a copy of the report to take with me to the Social Security office. (She told me later that she had sent the report from his testing for a second opinion, and the other doctor agreed with her results.)

I went to the Social Security office and applied for Ken's disability. It took several days of telephone calls, answering all of the questions, and sending a copy of my Power of Attorney. They were very helpful, and with Dr. Pepper's letter, his disability approval was expedited rather quickly.

PSALMS 13: 1-6

HOW LONG WILT, THOU FORGET ME, O LORD? FOREVER? HOW LONG WILT THOU HIDE THY FACE FROM ME! THOSE THAT TROUBLED ME REJOICE WHEN I'M MOVED I WILL SING UNTO THE LORD, BECAUSE HE HAVE DEALT BOUNTIFULLY WITH ME

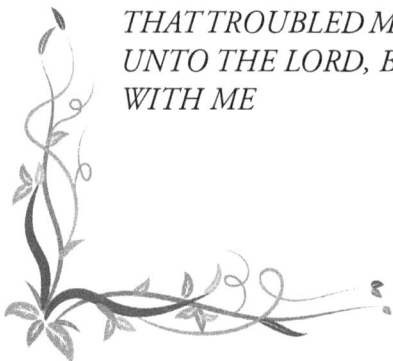

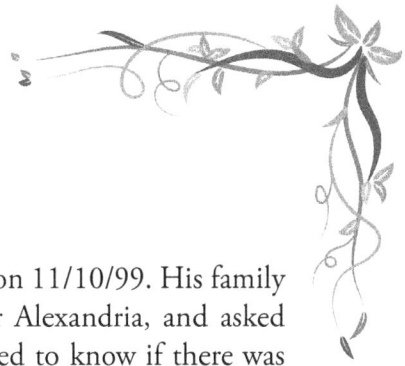

11/10/99

Ken had an appointment with Dr. Weaver on 11/10/99. His family had not been supportive, so I called his sister Alexandria, and asked her to meet us at the doctor's office. She wanted to know if there was something she wouldn't want to hear. I told her possibly. I felt sure Dr. Weaver would discuss his diagnosis at length, and could answer any of her questions.

Ken rode with Alexandria, and her husband, and I met them there. When I walked in, she and Ken were already seated, and I could tell Alexandria was already upset. I felt that it was because we were in a psychiatrist's office. Dr. Weaver asked Alexandria if she and the family had noticed any difference in Ken. She crossed her arms, sort of laughed and said, "Polly, I'm sorry, but I have to say what I feel." She then told Dr. Weaver, "Frankly, we don't know very much about this situation. For whatever reason, Polly has told us very little about what's going on. Every time one of us calls, she tells bad things he did, and we don't want to hear it. Besides, we all have trouble with remembering." He looked at her and asked, "Is yours as bad as Kenneth's?"

When we walked out to the car, Alexandria was so angry with me. She said, "I don't believe Kenneth has Alzheimer's. I believe something's wrong, but it's not Alzheimer's." I asked her to go back and talk with the doctor. She said, "There's no need. All he knows is what you and Kenneth have told him. It'll come out on down the road. She had made the same comments in the doctor's office.

I had asked his siblings to read the book, "The 36 Hour Day," when he was diagnosed, and they didn't think it necessary. I could tell she was really upsetting Ken. He'd look at her, and then look at me. I kept my voice even so as not to upset him even more. I wanted to take him home, but had only asked off from work long enough for the appointment.

PSALMS 121:1,2

I WILL LIFT UP MINE EYES UNTO THE HILLS, FROM WHICH COMETH MY HELP. MY HELP COMETH FROM THE LORD, WHICH MADE HEAVEN AND EARTH.

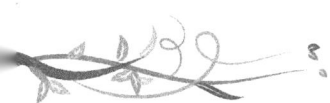

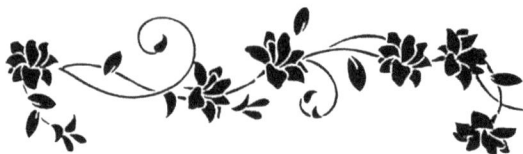

NO ESCAPE

The walls are closing around me;
no windows, no doors
no day, no night, no light.
There is so much hurt buried deep
as my life is being smothered,
without, and within.
I don't fully understand why the
innocent suffers from someone
else's sin.
Life goes on even when the ice is thin.
Oh, Lord, heal my breaking heart,
and comfort loved ones whom
I hold dear.

12/10/99

03/28/00

Ken enjoyed singing in the choir at church. I played the organ, and the way he was seated, he could see me. We attended as long as I could help dress him. The last cantata he sang in, I stood beside him on the back row, and tried to help him hold the book. He would flip the pages back and forth, and never missed a word. It was amazing. Many times as we were leaving church on Sunday, he would ask me a person's name. They had no idea that he didn't know their name. He would say, "I know that I know them, but I can't remember their name."

For the last three months Ken keeps saying that he's so tired he doesn't want to do anything. He'll sleep a lot on Saturday and Sunday. Labor Day he said, "I had planned to go to the farm, and bush hog, but I don't feel like it."

I casually mentioned to Ken, that his tiredness could be coming from his depression and the Alzheimer's. (One of his doctors had told me that he was not only dealing with depression, which was bad enough, but also, the Alzheimer's.) Ken refused to discuss anything from his childhood. I asked him why he didn't want to talk about his childhood, and he said, "It was really bad, I don't want to remember."

(Ken told me at a later date, that he had been sexually molested as a child. When he would recall some of his childhood, there was a jump from one incident to another, which included a period of five years. This was later determined to have occurred approximately between the ages of 8 and 13. *It made me very angry that no one had tried to help him in getting counseling.* One of his doctors said that if he could have counseled him when he was younger, he could have helped him, but it's too late now.) **Refer to page 42, dated 9/28/96**

Ken took his bath, shaved, dressed, and went out the door. I thought he had gone out to smoke. When he didn't come back in, I looked for him, and his truck was gone. He came home about 3:30 p.m. When he came in the door, he was very pale. I asked, "Where have you been?" In the same breath, I'm asking, "What's wrong?" He said, "I've been around the world and back. I got lost. I went to Walnut Cove to see Doris. I wound up in Kernersville, and had to stop two or three times to find out where I was."

(Doris is Ken's 1st cousin on his mama's side. If I have understood correctly; after Evelyn and Ken were no longer alive, all of Evelyn's siblings had Alzheimer's. Doris and all her siblings, also had Alzheimer's.)

When there has been ANY TYPE OF PHYSICAL, MENTAL, OR SEXUAL ABUSE, there will be a difficult path ahead for anyone involved. This usually, not always, follows a pattern. There are different reasons someone seeks a doctor's help. When some type of neurological or sexual problems enter the equation, this information should be shared. This is of immense importance to correctly diagnose, and treatment. The book UNDERSTANDING SEXUAL ABUSE, AUTHOR TIM HEIN, is a well written documentary of he and his wife's own experience.

ROMANS 12: 19, 21

DEARLY BELOVED, AVENGE NOT YOURSELVES, BUT RATHER GIVE PLACE UNTO WRATH; FOR IT IS WRITTEN, VENGEANCE IS MINE, SAITH THE LORD. BE NOT OVERCOME OF EVIL, BUT OVERCOME EVIL WITH GOOD.

HEBREWS 11:10

FOR WE KNOW HIM THAT SAID, VENGEANCE BELONGETH UNTO ME I WILL RECOMPENSE, SAITH THE LORD. IT IS A FEARFUL THING TO FALL INTO THE HANDS OF THE LIVING GOD.

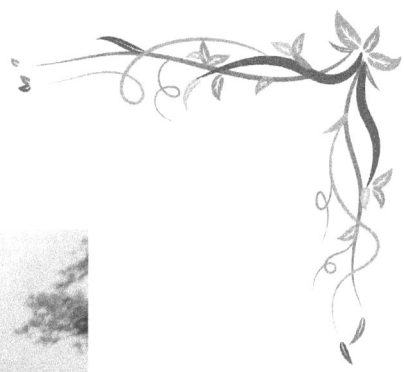

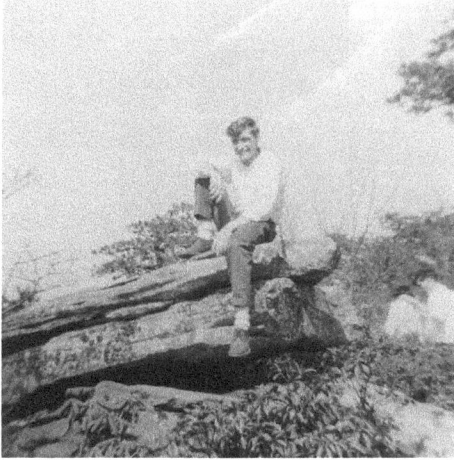

Made in the pinnacle of the Pilot Knob in the Spring of 1967.

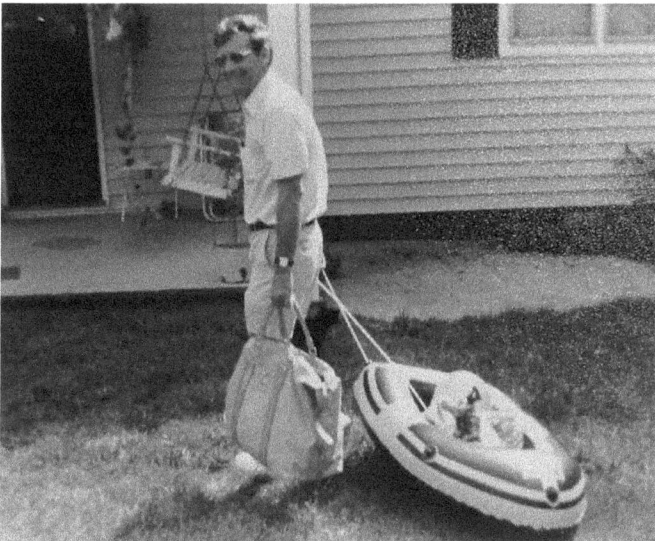

Coming home from White Lake – 1987

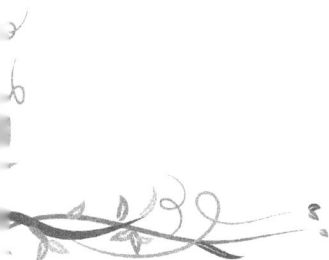

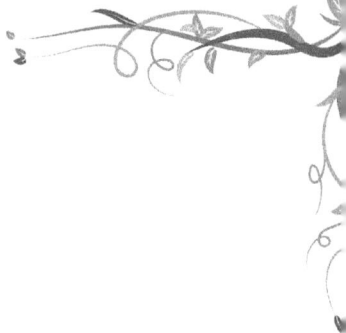

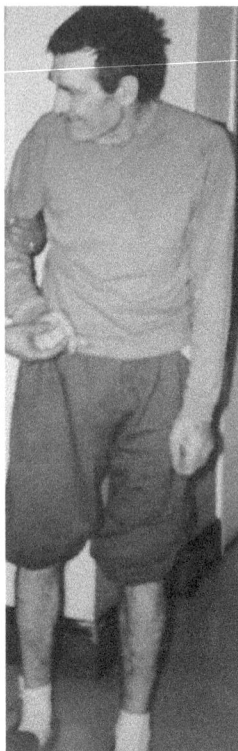

Ken in a sweatshirt – 2005
Sweatshirt and sweatpants or dress requirements for the
stage of Alzheimer's no other colors were available.

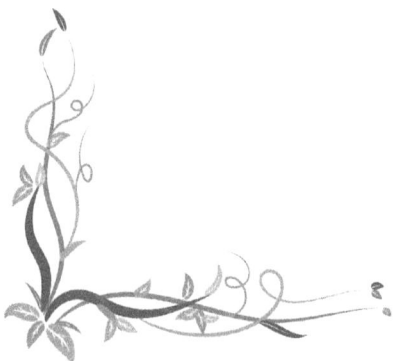

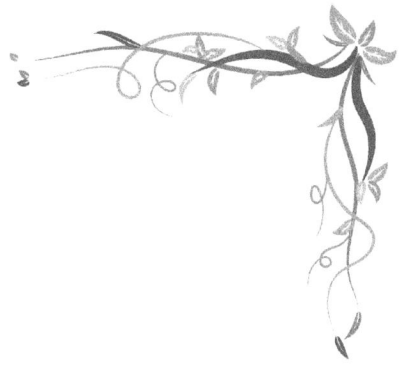

05/05/00

When I came home from work, Ken had this anxious expression on his face. I asked if he was OK. and he said, "Yes." As I kept talking to him, I noticed dried blood on his elbow and arm. He said his shoe had caught over the strip at the kitchen door, and he fell down the step. I cleaned his arm, and applied antibiotic. He wouldn't let me put an ice pack on it for the swelling. It's very difficult to decide if I should take him to the doctor.

05/13/00

After breakfast this morning, Ken went back to bed. I took Daddy to Mt. Airy, and when I came back Ken was still in the bed. When he got up, he ate lunch. Lots of times he'll say, I'm not hungry, but will eat when I put the food on the table.

Later, we worked out in the yard. Ken worked really hard, but he'd wait for me to instruct him. I'm doing things that I've never done before.

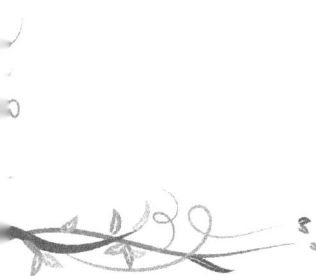

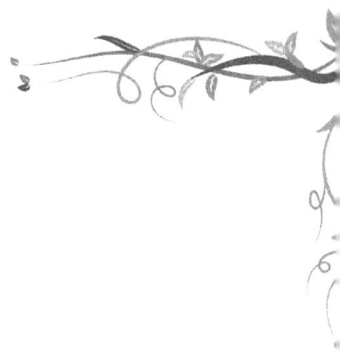

05/14/00

On the way to Sunday School this morning, Ken kept turning the pages of his Sunday School quarterly. I folded it to the right page, and told him that I needed to practice my music, and for him to go to the class. He made about two steps, and stopped. He asked me, "Where is our Sunday School class?" He stayed with me while I practiced. When we came home, he ate a good lunch, and slept all afternoon.

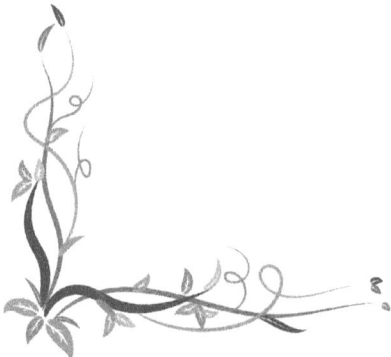

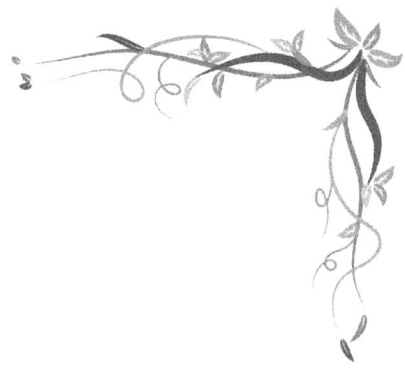

08/12/00

Ken became angry with me because he wanted to go to the farm. I reminded him, that Dr. Weaver had told him he wasn't supposed to drive anymore, because of his memory problems, and the seizures. He said, "I know how to drive, and I've not had any more seizures since taking my medicine." I told him that I'd take him to the farm. He said, "If I can't drive, I'm not going. If I'm not allowed to do anything, I may as well shoot myself. I'm not as bad as you all think I am." I fixed our lunch, and he refused to eat.

When I left to go get Dad at Mount Airy, he said, "I'll be gone when you get back. I'm going to the farm." I told him when I returned, we'd go to the farm. He looked at me, and said, "I don't like you." When I came home, I told him that I was going to the farm, and if he wanted to go, to come on. He was alright by the time we got there, and seemed fine.

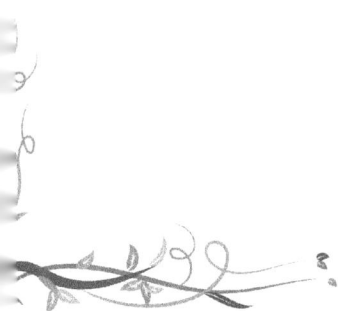

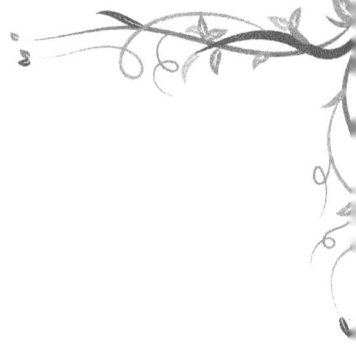

08/18/00

When I got home from work and having my hair cut, I could tell Ken was upset. He ate, and then sat in his recliner. I was walking past him, and he said, "You'd better get my truck fixed." I didn't answer, and he asked me again, "Did you hear me? I said you'd better get my truck fixed." I told him that I hadn't had the time. He then said, "Are you ready to die?" I said, "I am, why?" He said, "If you don't fix the truck so I can drive it, I'll kill you!" I asked how he planned to do that. He said, "I'll shoot you, or crush your head with a rock. You know I have some big ones on the carport." I asked, "What will you do with both vehicles?" His reply was, "I'll drive both of them." (I have been told that someone with Alzheimer's can't think to follow through with their threats, but I can't help but wonder.)

I hid the ammunition. His doctor told me to be ready to leave home at a minute's notice. It's like walking on eggshells. (Another doctor who is our friend, but had nothing to do with his diagnosis, told me not to turn my back on him.) As his caregiver, I'm not supposed to let him know if I'm sad or upset, because he will react accordingly.

In the beginning I would leave sandwiches in the refrigerator for Ken, but as time went on, he would not have eaten all day that I could tell. He spent a lot of time with our neighbors across the road. Frank would take him for rides to get him out of the house, and they would watch TV together. Frank and Grace would watch for him, and help him cross the road to their house, and then back home. His cousin, Kelly, who lived close by would stop and visit with Ken while I was at work. Kelly had a brother, P.W. who came to see him, and they went for a ride. When I came home, and Ken wasn't home, I panicked. About that time, they pulled in the driveway. They were both laughing. He had such a good time. I was thankful that P.W. had taken the time to do that.

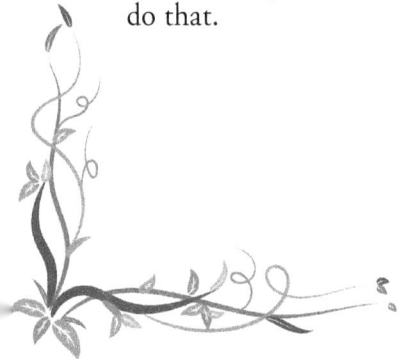

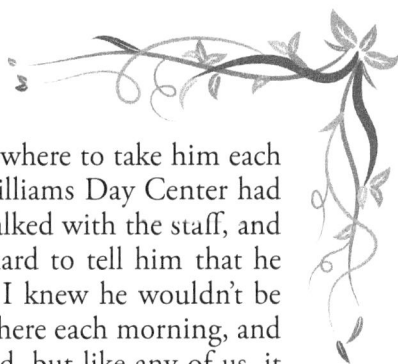

The time had come that I had to find somewhere to take him each day while I worked. The Elizabeth and Tab Williams Day Center had been recommended. I visited the facility, and talked with the staff, and felt that he would be in good hands. It was hard to tell him that he would no longer be staying at home, because I knew he wouldn't be happy in a strange location. I would take him there each morning, and go back to get him each afternoon. He adjusted, but like any of us, it wasn't like being at home.

10/13/00

I went to the Day Center to get Ken. As he came from the back, he gave me one of his "I'm upset" looks. When he got in the car, I told him that I had an appointment to get my hair cut. He didn't say anything. He was very quiet until I exited at King, and he said, "I'm not going with you to get your hair cut. I asked if he wanted me to take him to his brother's, and he said, "Nope. I'll just walk home. I'm not waiting for you."

When we got to the beauty shop, he refused to get out. His niece, who also cuts my hair, tried to get him to come in. She said he talked like a child when she asked him what was wrong. He said he couldn't tell her.

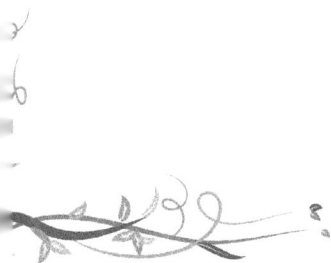

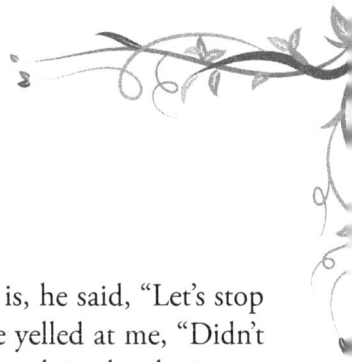

As we went by the garage where Ken's truck is, he said, "Let's stop and take the truck home." I kept driving, and he yelled at me, "Didn't you hear what I said?" I said, "Yes." I tried to explain that he is not allowed to drive, and he grabbed the gear stick, and tried to push it to reverse. I caught it just in time, and he turned it loose. He was very angry with me. He did eat supper, but was very subdued.

****

I cleaned house, and left at 10:00 a.m. to go to work. I got home about 3:00 p.m. He ate a sandwich with me. I tried to get him to go with me to get groceries, but he refused. When I came back, I went to see my 91 year old Dad, who was home from the hospital after having a massive heart attack. When I got back, I cooked supper, and Ken wouldn't eat, and wouldn't take his medicine. Later I went to bed. I had put his depression pill in with the other medicine. When I got up Sunday morning, he had taken all of his medicine.

****

He later talked with his sister, Delight, and began putting me down, and called me a Hammerhead. He told her that the doctor and I thought we knew more than he did, and that I'd taken his truck and keys away. He told her if he didn't get his truck back, he would start tearing up some things, and he'd tear up some butt. He then said real loud, "Polly, did you hear that? I've done good to hold my anger, and I'd better get my truck back. I'll make them pay, you just wait and see. I'll be glad when I get to Heaven 'cause Polly and Dr. Weaver won't be there to tell me what to do."

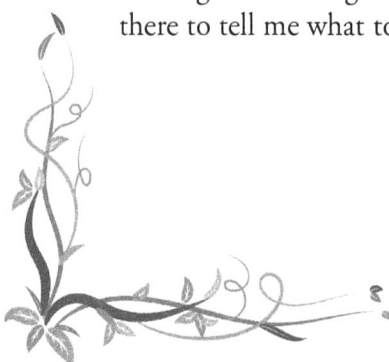

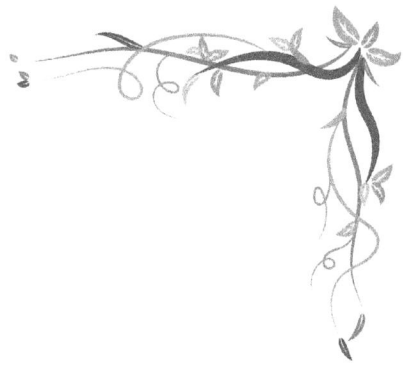

2/06/00

There has been a definite change in Ken the last month. He is now taking four to five Risperdal daily and three Depakote daily. Last Tuesday, he had a seizure as I was getting ready to take Daddy to his two doctor appointments. I called Dr. Crowell. He said to come to his office to pick up a lab request, for some blood work. He called a couple of days later, and left a message for me to give Ken four Depakote, rather than three. He is no longer taking Aricept as it doesn't seem to be working any more. He is taking 2000IU vitamin E daily.

****

Ken will walk around in the house with a cigarette in his hand, and reach in his pack for another one. Then he becomes confused as to what to do with them. He doesn't smoke in the house. He is having trouble completing sentences. He says just enough for me to question if he means thus and so. He walks slowly, or shuffles, and never gets in a hurry. He will have on his clothes, and look for them. He misplaces his cap and glasses often. I help him get his clothes together. He keeps asking the same question over, and over. He can't tell the time anymore, and he asks often, "What day is it, and what month?"

****

Most of the time, I cut his meat for him, or he will hold it with his fingers. Some times he tries to use a knife rather than a fork. He seems to be having trouble breathing, and it sounds as if he has asthma. He is not as aggressive as he was at one time. I don't know if it's the Risperdal, or just another stage of Alzheimer's.

****

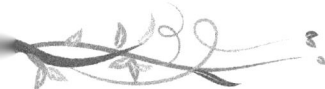

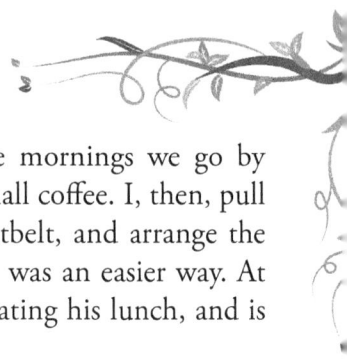

I now help him fasten his seat belt. Some mornings we go by McDonalds, and get him a gravy biscuit, and small coffee. I, then, pull off to the side, and put a napkin under his seatbelt, and arrange the container, so he can eat as we ride. I wish there was an easier way. At least, I know that he's not home by himself, is eating his lunch, and is not by himself.

****

A couple of weeks ago, I had been out for a while, and when I returned I sat down on the couch. He looked at me, and asked, "Where's the children?" That is the first time that I knew he did not know me, or had me confused with someone else.

****

He is having trouble knowing what he wants to eat. He'll say, "I'm hungry, but I don't know what I want." When I suggest something, he may say no, and want to know what else we have, etc.

****

He'll start to say something and stop. Sunday, he said, "It's frustrating not to be able to remember what I was going to say." He may forget to do something, go in the other room, and then ask me why he went in there.

****

There are times that we'll be watching TV or talking about something, and out of nowhere, he'll make an observation that has nothing to do with the situation.

****

Saturday, Daddy and I went to Joy Ranch, which is a children's home. We stopped and picked up supper on our way home. Ken threw

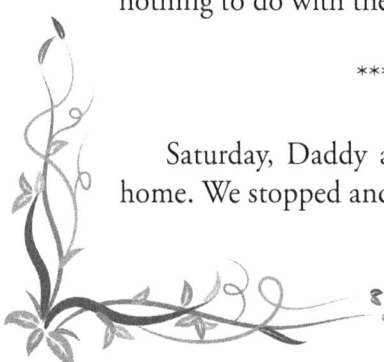

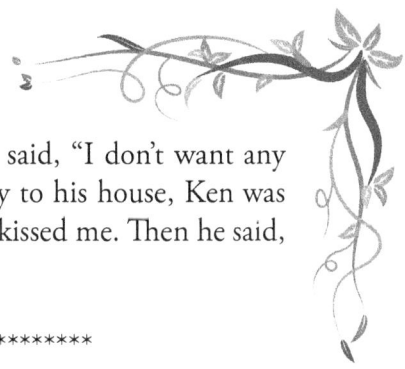

the take-out box of food across the table, and said, "I don't want any of that junk." When I got ready to take Daddy to his house, Ken was outside smoking. I walked over to him, and he kissed me. Then he said, "You are a snake, you know that?"

****

Ken had trouble remembering Christmas. He would hear advertisements on T.V., and then he'd ask, "When is Christmas?" Sometimes he'd think Christmas had already been.

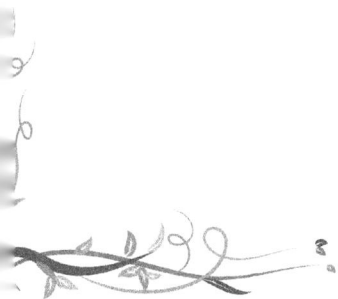

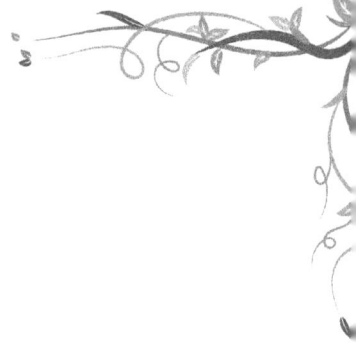

04/02/02

The Day Care talked with me at length, and I was told that they felt it is definitely time to put Ken in an assisted living facility. They recommended Brighton Gardens. I made an appointment and talked with the manager about the cost, and toured the Alzheimer's unit. It was clean, well-staffed, and the residents appeared to be well cared for. We agreed on a date to bring Ken in. This was one of the hardest things I've ever had to do. How do you tell someone that they no longer will be coming home? I was advised to not go see him for at least two weeks in order for him to adjust to his new surroundings. I couldn't do that. For an Alzheimer's person, fifteen minutes can seem like forever, but at the same time, they may not remember what took place five minutes ago.

I'd go by when I got off work and take him out to eat, and spend time with him. He'd always cry when I would have to leave. There was no way for him to understand. He was crazy about Wendy's Frosties. His sister, Susie, would take him, once a week for a long time, to get him one. He thoroughly enjoyed this.

There are so many things about Alzheimer's that we don't understand. It is a very cruel disease. Ken's room-mate fell out of his bed one night. When the staff was doing their routine check, they found Ken standing over him. Ken had pulled the blanket off his bed, and laid it over his room-mate. There were times that Ken would go get the manager. He couldn't tell her by words, but she could tell by his actions. He seemed to understand what she would say, and then he'd take her where something had happened.

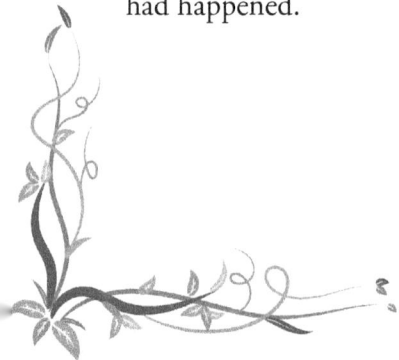

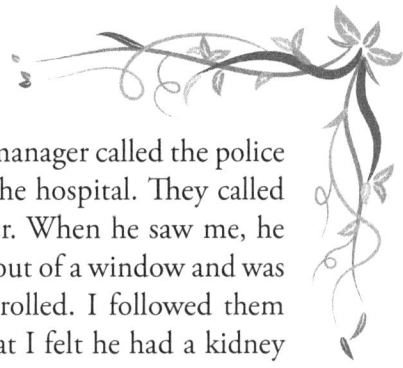

There was one episode with Ken where the manager called the police to calm Ken down, and EMS to take him to the hospital. They called me, and by the time I arrived, Ken was quieter. When he saw me, he reached for me. They said he had tried to jump out of a window and was running back and forth, and couldn't be controlled. I followed them to the hospital, and tried to tell the doctors that I felt he had a kidney stone, but I was just wasting my breath. He had kidney stones in the past. They looked at me as if I was crazy.

Ken was admitted to the psychiatry floor because of the Alzheimer's. While he was there, he had a Gran mall seizure that lasted twenty minutes. I'm glad I didn't see that. It's my understanding that when someone has this type for this long, that it can be fatal. The doctors were there and observed him. The day he was discharged and sent back to Brighton Gardens, he passed blood as he urinated. The manager and I both had felt the same, as to what was wrong with him, and we were right. How sad. He did the only thing he knew to do, and the doctors wouldn't listen.

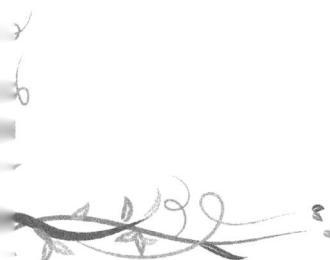

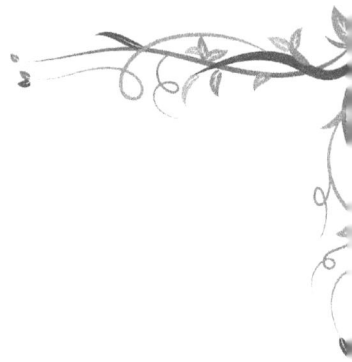

I haven't written anything in a long time in reference to Ken's Alzheimer's. It has been a downhill battle all the way. He almost died with Pancreatitis while he was still at Brighten Gardens.

Ken was sent by an ambulance to the emergency room at a local hospital three times in less than 24 hours. During this time, Ken was writhing from so much pain. (Stressful situation) I kept asking for medication to ease the pain and anxiety.

They would not administer, but I was repeatedly told to keep him still! That was impossible under ordinary circumstances; much less, for someone with Alzheimer's. Ken was lying on a gurney that was higher than I. Ken was much stronger than I; yet, I was expected to keep him still! *The doctor decided to review the blood work drawn from the three previous visits.* Ken was then diagnosed with Pancreatitis, and was put on morphine.

The doctor said Ken would have to be on clear IV's for a few days in order to flush the poison from his system. He also said that if the poison was already in his system, it would just be a matter of time before he died.

Even though he doesn't have any quality life now, it was a shock to hear. I was told when he was diagnosed with Alzheimer's that, medically, he would probably only live five years.

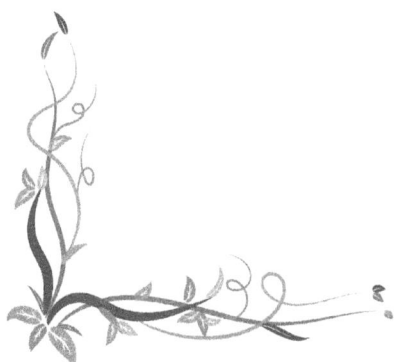

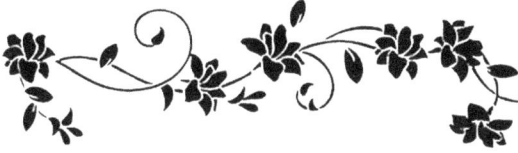

I NEED SOMEONE

What can I say?
What can I do?
My world is so empty without you.
I feel so lonely in the middle of the night,
needing someone to hold me tight.
I need someone with whom to share my dreams
no matter how trivial they may be.
My life is in a whirlwind with the road
in the future looking mighty dim.
Sometimes it seems that I'm under the ground
shoveling out a load of coal;
deeper and deeper I seem to go.
When I look back there's an empty space,
but when I see where I've been,
there's a peace that settles in.
In my lifetime, will there be
someone who will love only me?
That's for God to know and
for me to wait and see…

07/25/03

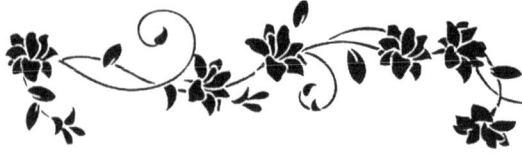

PLEASE HELP ME

I bowed my head in despair
as I cried out unto the lord,
"Please help me!
Show me the way You'd have me go.
Tell me what I need to do."
It seemed no answer would come through.
Then, in a quiet voice
I heard, "Be still and wait upon the Lord."
I am so frightened, and oh, so lonely.
The Lord reminded me,
"Put your trust in Me, and
I will supply your every need."
My Lord, I have to depend on You
to see me through,
as there is nothing else that I can do.

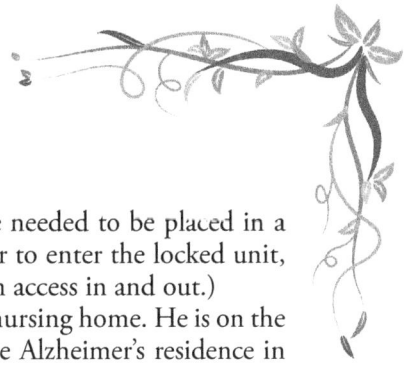

01/01/04

The doctor who diagnosed Ken, stated that he needed to be placed in a locked unit, for his and others protection. (In order to enter the locked unit, the person has to know the code in order to have an access in and out.)

When Ken left the hospital, he went to a local nursing home. He is on the Alzheimer's floor. (Some nursing home do not have Alzheimer's residence in a separate unit.) He is still aware enough to know what is happening to him, and he is frightened, as he can't control it.

(By this time, I was emotionally and physically wiped out. I was incapable of being attentive to him.) I was out of work with Chronic Depression and Anxiety for 6 months, but disability denied. They stated that I could have taken a less stressful job, or worked part time. How do you do that when you can't get out of the bed to take a bath? We have spent all of our saved monies, his retirement pension, and sold our 18 acre farm, in order to live and pay for his care. It's been hard to make such major decisions alone. I never mentioned these things to Ken, as it would have confused him.

During this time, my Dad was moved into a different nursing home. My brother took care of his needs, and paperwork. I don't have the words to describe how I felt. I was a Daddy's girl, and I wanted to be there for him. We had always been very close. I went to see him as often as I could, and lots of time it might be 9:00 p.m. or 10:00 p.m. If he was asleep, I'd just sit and hold his hand.

Since Ken arrived at the nursing home, he has been walking almost constantly. The staff who puts him to bed has shared with me that they will put on his pajamas, see that he is in bed, and covered up. As they go out the door, he will come out behind them.

Each resident in the nursing home was given a guardian (an employee) who I was to go to if there were any problems. In the past months I have spoken to Ken's guardian about his clothes being wrinkled, and looked as if he had slept in them. Also, his clothes were mixed up with his roommate's. At least fifteen pairs of nice socks with Ken's name on them have been lost (either both or one of a set). I don't have the receipts, so they won't reimburse me. It's the same with his pants and shirts. I have asked the staff several times about his socks, and they say it's the Laundry's fault.

One of his sisters became upset with me when I stated I wasn't buying him any more socks for someone else to wear. She bought him some, and wrote his name on them, but within a week, they were gone.

I have finally had to decide that if all of Ken's needs were put in a basket, other things such as his body hygiene, food, medicine, to name a few, would take priority. I insisted that he have on socks and shoes, even if the socks didn't match. Since he has been here, a coat that he'd only worn twice disappeared; shirts and pants that matched also disappeared. Since I don't have receipts for all of this, the facility won't replace these, either.

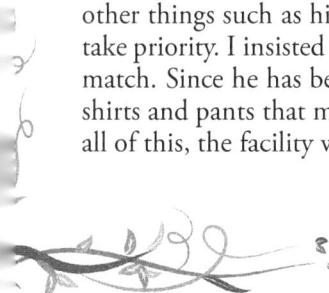

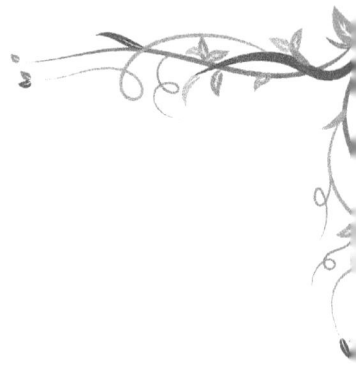

11/19/04

I talked with Ken's new guardian. She assured me that his face, and neck would be shaved, and that his hair would be kept clean. She also assured me that someone from outside would teach the nurses and CNA's how to work with Dementia residents, beginning December 1, 2004.

I told her that Ken's niece, Lewana, and I came to see Ken Saturday evening to cut his hair, and I knew it hadn't been washed for several days. Lewana said she could smell oil while she was cutting it. The guardian said she would tell the CNA's not to put oil conditioner on Ken's hair.

I told her that four of the residents were sitting in the hallway close to the Nurses Station when Lewana and I got off the elevator. We could smell an unpleasant odor, and one of the residents using a walker kept walking around us. When we left at least an hour or more, later, she hadn't been changed, and we could still smell an odor in the hallway. One of the residents only had on a shirt, and a Depend.

Ken went from walking constantly, to him being found sitting on the floor in the hallway, or lying in someone's bed. Wherever he was when he became tired, was where he would sit down. His favorite place was at the end of the hallway on the right. The sun would shine in the window in the afternoon. He was often found sitting in a chair in front of the window, asleep. There wouldn't be anyone else in the room.

When he first came here, he would go in the last room on the left, and the resident there would get so upset with him. When Ken was at Brighten Gardens, his room was the last one on the left. I'm sure this is where he thought he was going.

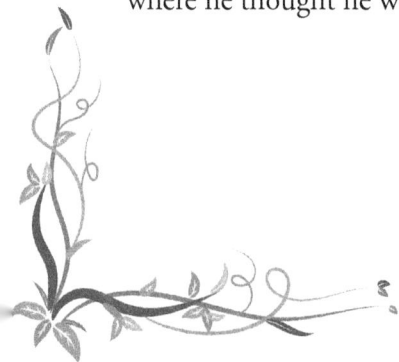

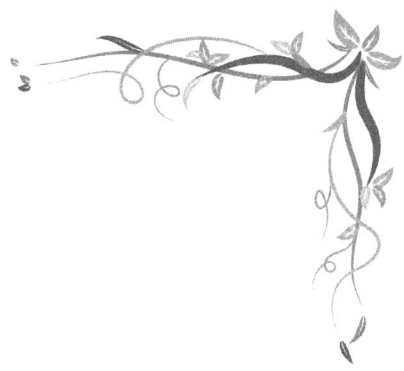

11/22/04

When I went to see Ken today, he was sitting in the dining room with The Activity Director, who had fed him, and she was feeding another resident. She is the only one whom I'm aware of who has had special training for Dementia. She is very good at her job.

The nurses and staff are constantly being sent to another floor. There is no consistency, and anyone with Alzheimer's training will tell you that consistency is of top priority.

Ken had his shoes on, but no socks. One of the staff told me that as long as a resident had on one or the other that it was alright. The floors in the hallway are most always dirty. Ken was halfway shaved, and his hair was not clean. I reiterated to her that he is to have socks and shoes on at the same time. The activity director was not the one who dressed him. **It's like talking to a wall.**

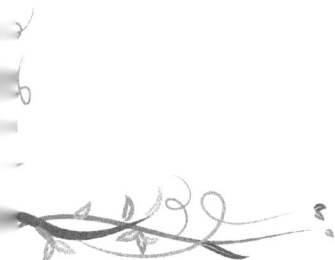

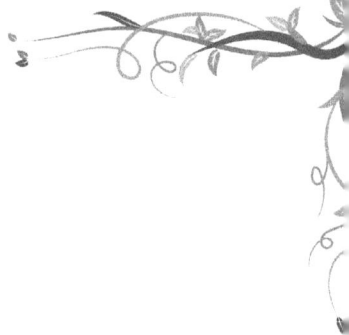

11/23/04

I went to see Ken today, and he was asleep in a chair in the dining room. He hadn't been shaved, no socks on, and his hair dirty. This was about 2:30 p.m. I had brought him some new clothes. His guardian had suggested that I get sweatpants, and pull over shirts. His name has been put on all of his clothes. I went to his room to hang them up, and his clothes were mixed with a resident's who was a former roommate. His new roommate is also named Kenneth. He wears a large size, and a medium is too big for Ken. Today, Ken had on a large pair of pants.

I went to the nurse's desk and asked who had dressed him today. The first shift nurse said she would find out. She also said that Ken didn't have on socks today, because he slapped the CNA, and that was also the reason he wasn't shaved. I understand that at times Ken can be combative, but there are eight hours on first shift, and eight hours on second shift.

When residents are fed, bibs aren't used, and residents who try to feed themselves will get food all over their clothes. This is not their fault that they aren't changed. I've noticed quite often when the CNA'S start to change Ken's Depend, or turn him over in the bed, they don't all talk to him. It frightens him, as it catches him unaware.

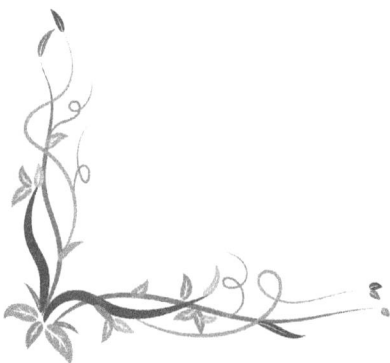

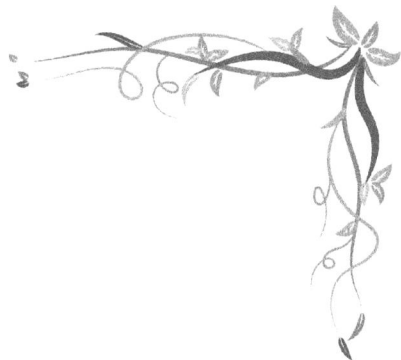

11/24/04

I went to see Ken about 3:00 p.m. His clothes were all mixed up with his room-mate, again. I told his guardian. He had been shaved, but still not around his lips and neck. His hair still felt and looked dirty. He didn't seem to be feeling well. CNA said that he didn't get up until 11:00 a.m. and when she tried to feed him, she had to wake him up. He only ate half of his food, and went back to sleep.

The physical therapist came to his room, and he was sitting in his wheelchair asleep. She said she had checked on him two or three times to walk him, and he had been asleep. We woke him enough to walk a few steps with her help. He barely woke up enough to try to drink a little of his milkshake. He usually will drink all of it.

The kitchen sent up peanut butter nabs <u>again</u> without liquid of any kind. We had to sit him back in his wheelchair. I asked the nurse about him sleeping so much. She said, "He's not sleeping, he just has his eyes closed." I looked at her, and she gave me a look that dared me to question her.

Ken is now on a wheelchair. He has gone from walking, to staggering as he is losing muscle control. The wheelchair is equipped with a lap-buddy to keep him from getting out, or falling out, if he goes to sleep. I had to sign for the lap—buddy, but I had to think of his safety.

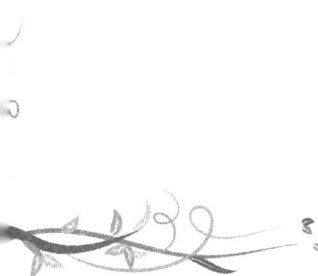

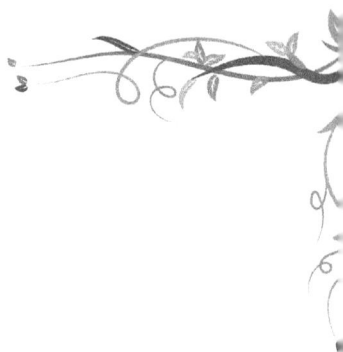

11/26/04

The cafeteria sent up snacks about 2:00 p.m. They had sent nabs for Ken. He doesn't have any upper teeth. He had an upper plate, but the staff kept finding his teeth in other rooms, in flower pots, etc., so I took them home. He tried and tried to bite the nabs, but couldn't. I finally took them from him, and broke into smaller pieces. He would chew on it for a while. I asked the CNA, if she would get me some juice, or water. She said she didn't have any juice, but she brought a half pint of milk. Ken reached for it, and I let him drink as he ate. I feel as if he doesn't get enough to drink.

The clothes in his closet were all mixed up again. I straightened them up. When I went downstairs, I knocked on the nursing director's office door. I told her about the clothes, and she called Laundry to come to her office. She asked him if there was something he could do, and he said he thought so. At one time there was a plastic ring between each resident's clothes. He would get one for Ken's room. The nurse suggested maybe one of the resident's was doing this. I told her I didn't think so. I'm finding this too often. She said she had seen a lady coming down the hall with a roommate's clothes. She appeared to feel that I was making a big deal out of it.

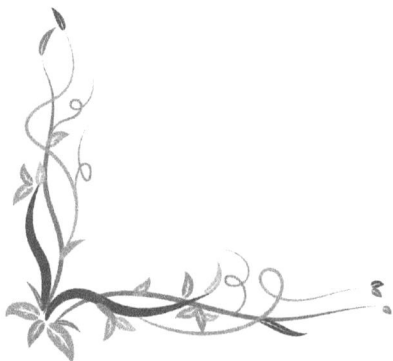

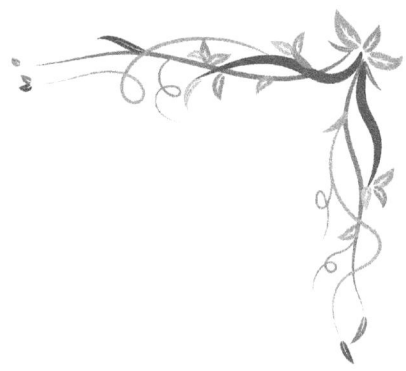

11/30/04

I went to see Ken at 4:45 p.m. I carried him food from the K & W Restaurant. He ate very well. His hair was clean, but he wasn't shaven. His bed had been lowered, but the foot was higher than his head. I would like to put the staff who does this, in the same position for a day, and see if they like it.

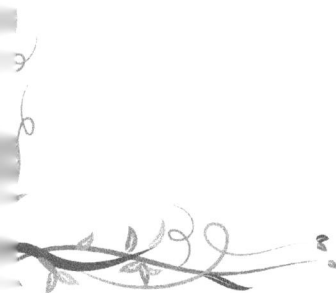

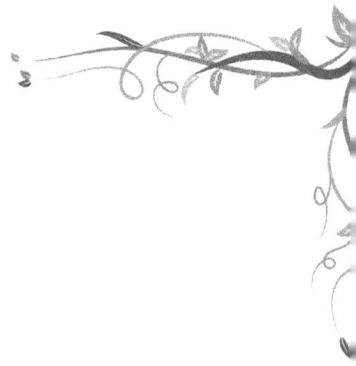

01/06/05

I visited Ken and things still have not improved. I went to the office on ground floor, Ken's guardian was working. The secretary paged her. When she returned the call she was in a meeting. She didn't say that she would call, and didn't ask for my number.

01/07/05

I left a message for Ken's guardian to call me at work. I carried my cell phone with me most of the morning, and then left it on my desk. Someone told me that my desk phone was ringing. I looked to see if I had a message, and there wasn't one. I was expecting two other calls, but I called her back, just in case it was her. She said it was, and I said, "You didn't leave me a message." Her response was, "Well, it wasn't that important, I was going to call back later." My response was, "I have been expecting your call, and two others, and they were all important."

I then asked her the status on training for dementia care. She wasn't sure, and then I repeated what she said in November 22, 2004. She said, *"No, I said someone within the company would be doing the training, and we have many facilities. I don't know when they'll get to us."* I thought for a facility to advertise that they have an Alzheimer's unit that the employees would have to be trained appropriately. *Guess I was wrong.*

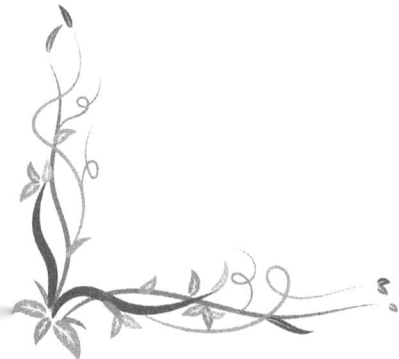

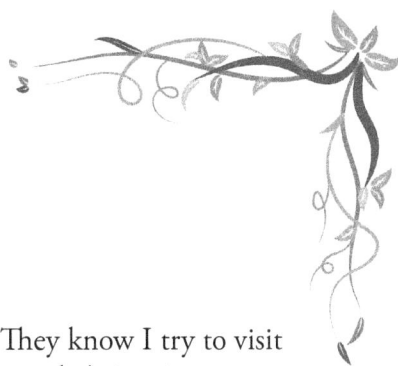

01/10/05

I went to see Ken today at a different time. They know I try to visit every day, but not the time. He had on someone else's jogging pants. They were too loose, and kept sliding down. He responded to his name today. He drank part of his milkshake, and then went on down the hall. He's learned to navigate well in his wheelchair.

When I entered the dining room, there was a hospital table on the left. A tray was on it with leftovers, and dirty dishes. I have seen this type of thing several times. It's unsanitary as some of the residents could walk by, and try to eat from them.

I went to Ken's room and four of his unmatched socks were laying on the floor behind the door. He had four pair of jogging pants. I took his slacks, folded them up, and brought them home. Unmatched shoes were lying on the floor. They have been there since Ken came last January. I took pictures.

Ken had been shaved, but had nicks all over his face. Someone shaved him with a regular razor, instead of his personal electric one. I get so frustrated I could scream if it would help any.

As Ken and I were walking down the hall, there was a broom and dustpan propped against the wall. One of the resident's was in a wheelchair, and it was caught against the trash containers setting out in the middle of the floor. I had clothes in one hand, and Ken's milkshake in the other. He picked up the broom trying to figure out what to do with it. As I was trying to get my camera a male CNA came up the hall. He took the broom and the dustpan, and propped them against the door to a room. I'm sure that took some thinking. What is considered a negligence?

The CNA handed Ken a pack of nabs, and he tried to put paper and all in his mouth. She said, "Maybe I better open them," and she handed him one. He doesn't know how to open them, and he can't bite them. I have seen one resident take food away from another resident. She should have been aware of the situation, but I get the feeling so often, that they don't really care.

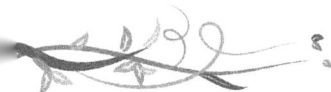

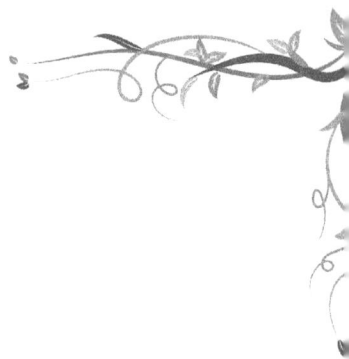

2/09/05

I went to a meeting about expectations for Ken. I asked again that he be given more water to drink. I also asked why Ken's nails, and hair stayed so dirty, and why he's not being shaved. I was told that sometimes he wouldn't let anyone shave him. I told her that I shouldn't have to ask for his nails to be cleaned.

I also told them that several times trays of food were left on tables, and residents would eat out of them. This really concerns me. She said they weren't supposed to be left unattended, and that this would be looked into. **Why had this not already been reported or resolved? Ken, or someone else could have eaten this sandwich and choked on the plastic!!!**

I asked if Ken could be given softer food, as he is having trouble chewing without his upper teeth. She said she would have his food pureed.

Evidently someone is not taking responsibility. It should be documented in the resident's chart and not in **print.**

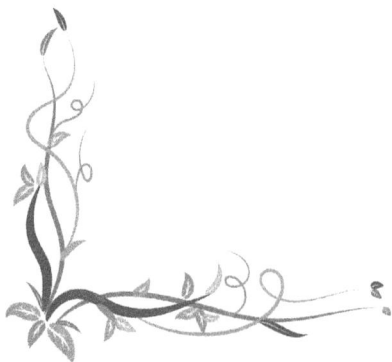

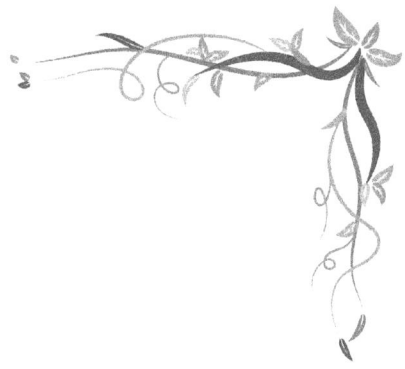

02/12/05

My friend Anne and I went to see Ken. When we got off the elevator we began to look for him. He wasn't in the dining room. We checked rooms where the door was open, but we didn't go in. We still couldn't find him. I told the nurse where we had looked. She and the CNA's began going into the rooms. After about twenty five minutes, a CNA hollered that he had found him. Ken was lying on the floor under the Activities desk asleep. **Why is he not looked after?**

His supper was delivered, and I fed him. He ate the food that was soft enough. His fingernails have been dirty. I clean them each time I come.

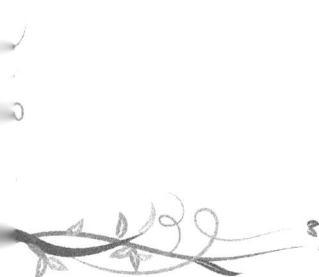

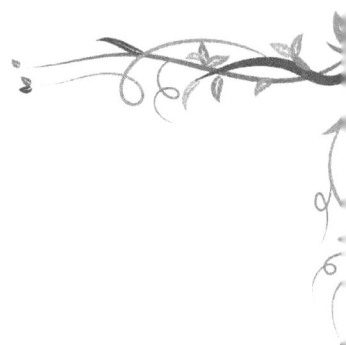

02/14/05

I went to see Ken. He was down the hall, and when the CNA told him that I was there, I heard him laugh, and he started up the hall. I met him with his Valentine card. When he saw the red envelope, he reached for it. He could have cared less about the card, but he hung on to the envelope for a long time.

I fed him his pureed supper. He was about half through when his sister, Susie, and her husband came to see him. He was excited. He kept looking at her, laughing, and tried to talk to her. He didn't eat quite all of his food, but drank a lot of liquid.

I went in his room, and under his bed near the wall was what looked like a lot of dried liquid, and a plastic glove. It was very unsanitary. There was a sandwich in plastic laying on the night table. I noticed a tray at the nurses' station. It had graham crackers with Ken's name on it with the time of 10:00 a.m. It was approximately 5:00 p.m. when I was there. If they don't feed him, he can't feed himself. The nurse said she would notify housekeeping to clean his floor.

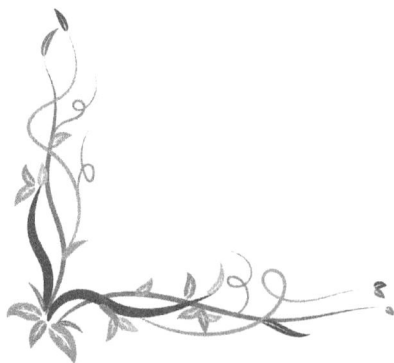

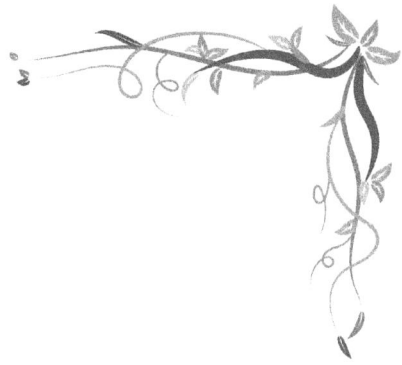

02/15/05

I called the nursing home this morning, and asked to speak to whoever is over housekeeping. I told him who I was. I told him that I was calling about housekeeping not cleaning the floors. He said, "I sent one of the boys up there, and he said it looked like urine, and he has gone to mop it up." I asked, "Why did you wait until this morning when it was found yesterday afternoon?" He said, "Housekeeping goes home at 3:00p.m." I asked, "If something like this happens anywhere, is it left until the next day?" He said, "Nurses and CNA's are supposed to clean it up." I was furious, and told him that is a shoddy way to run a business. I got the impression that it didn't bother him. I called back, and asked to speak to the administrator, and had to leave my name and number. He left me a message that he will be in his office tomorrow.

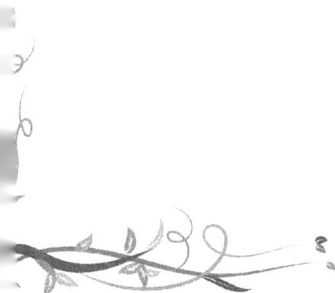

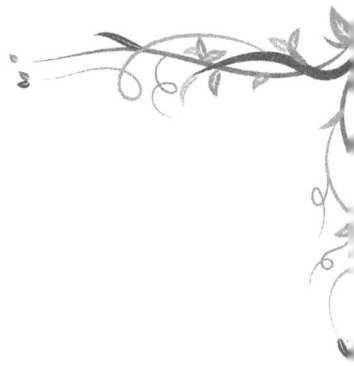

08/08/06

Ken didn't pay much attention to me as I entered his room, and talked to him. I proceeded to hang up his clothes. When I came back within his vision, he smiled and said "Hey there." It was as clear as he ever spoke, and just as quickly, he was somewhere else. He began to look upward, and his gaze moved around. He looked toward me, but it seemed he was seeing something other than me. He kept looking, and I just watched him. One time he frowned, sort of, as if he was really concentrating on what he was seeing. All at once, he said "Alf" which is the way he would say Ralph, now. I asked him if he had seen Ralph, and he didn't respond. This was a brother who died approximately two years ago. He has been gazing like this for about a week and a half.

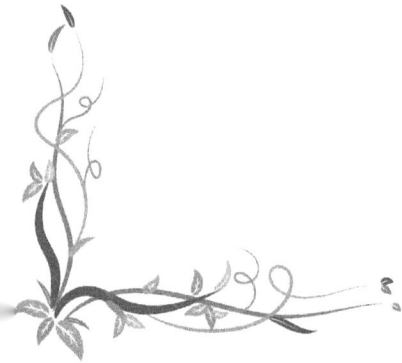

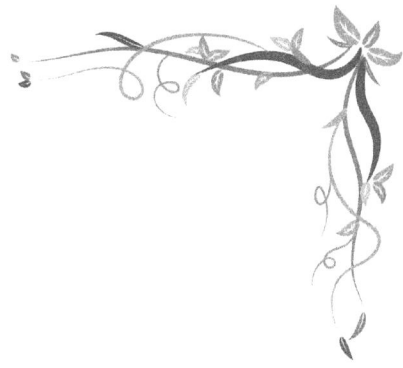

08/15/06

I went by the nursing home this morning on my way to work. I had planned to hang up Ken's clothes and go on to work. When I walked in he seemed to be in deep thought, and was looking around. I sat the bag on the floor and stood by his bed observing him. His eyes were big as saucers as he kept gazing from side to side as he looked upward. As he was looking, he said real strongly, "GO, GO!" I realized his chin was trembling a lot. I reached out, placed my hand on his cheek and chin, and said, "It's OK" All at once his hand went to his stomach, and he hollered, "OH!" His body then jerked real hard. He had reached for my hand, and was squeezing real hard, and seemed to be frightened.

Could this have been pertaining to earlier abuse or some intense pain from a kidney stone? I guess I'll never know. It hurts to watch him.

I stayed with him observing, then went to nurses station, called my supervisor and told her I felt I needed to stay with him a while longer. His breakfast was brought in, and I fed him. He drank some of his coffee through a straw, and some of his juice. He then began to strangle when he swallowed. I stopped giving it to him. At intervals, he would say something to me, but I couldn't understand him. After eating, he seemed to want to sleep, so I made sure he was comfortable, and left his room. I talked to his nurse, and left for work.

This afternoon, I had appointment to get a perm. When I left the beauty shop, it was about 7:30 p.m., so I went back to the nursing home. Ken seemed to be seeing someone or something again. He became restless, and I asked the CNA if she would turn him on his side, which she did. He seemed comfortable, so I left. This is so heartbreaking.

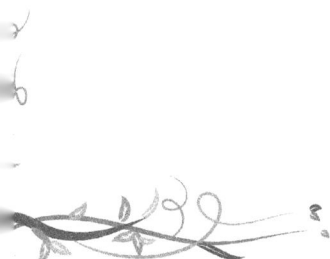

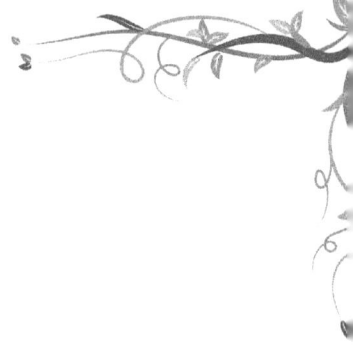

08/16-17/06

I went by to see Ken after work each day. On Wednesday, he was in the dining area with the CNA. She was trying to feed him, but he wouldn't open his mouth. He had drunk about 1/2 of his tea. I tried to get him to eat something. He did eat about 3 small spoons of food, but when he tried to drink his juice, he got strangled which scared him. He ate his ice cream, but barely opened his mouth enough for me to let ice cream slide into his mouth. He was so tired. The CNA put him to bed, and he was asleep by the time his head was on the pillow. On the 17th, he was basically the same as the 16th. The CNA said, "He ate all of his food, but got strangled on water. It will need to be thickened, but he drank his juice and milk without any problem."

08/23/06

Ken has been sticking his finger in his ear and he keeps moving his tongue around his last tooth in back on the left side. He acts as if it is hurting him. When I told him I would ask the nurse to give him something for the pain, he looked at me as if he knew what I was saying.

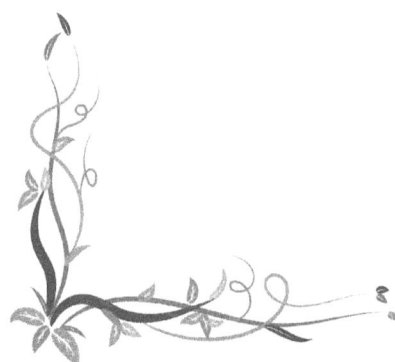

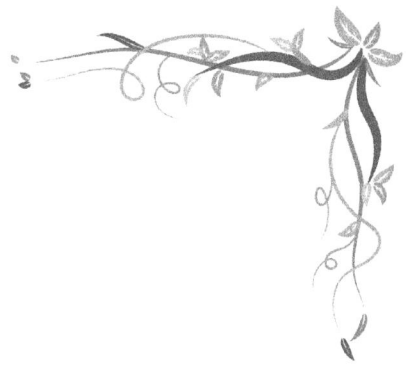

08/25/06

Craig Walker, the Chaplin with Hospice came to visit Ken. He had called me earlier, and asked questions about what he did at work and play. I told him that he built commercial dishwashers. For twenty-five years he had volunteered to umpire baseball and softball games.

When Mr. Walker came in, he took Ken's hand with his left hand and with his right hand, patted Ken on the shoulder, and kept rubbing his arm as he talked. He kept eye contact with Ken, and Ken acted as if he was mesmerized. When Mr. Walker began talking about building the dishwashers, Ken started talking back to him (in his language now). It's so sad to not know what he is saying, 'cause he tries so hard. Each time that Mr. Walker would say something, Ken would respond. When he talked about singing, Ken lit up, and jabbered some more. When he mentioned the umpiring, Ken laughed and really jabbered.

Mr. Walker said he would like to have communion with us, if that was alright with Ken, and Ken responded as if it was. We are to meet with Mr. Walker in the morning at 10:00. Before he left, he wanted to have prayer. He took Ken's left hand, and I took his right. Ken squeezed my hand during the prayer, and I felt he knew what was being said.

After Mr. Walker left, the CNA came in to take off Ken's shirt and put his nightgown on. He was propped up some in his bed. All at once, he sat straight up, and reached out both arms, as he was looking in front of him and up. He then sort of fell back on the bed and jerked his head toward me. It seemed he was in a transitional state. WOW!

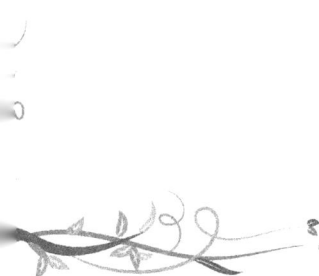

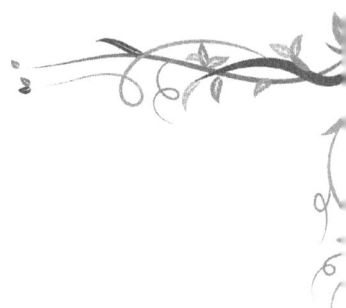

08/26/06

I got to the nursing home about 9:45 a.m., and Ken was sitting in the dining room. When I spoke to him, he didn't respond. He looked so tired and sleepy. I pushed him in his wheelchair out of the dining room, and the next thing I knew, he was slumped over the lap-buddy with his right hand hanging down beside his wheelchair. When Mr. Walker arrived, we went downstairs to an office where it would be quieter. The communion was very meaningful. We listened to a tape of Gold City singing a cappella. The first song was "His Name is Wonderful." As Mr. Walker talked and read the scripture, Ken kept trying to hold his head up, but he just couldn't. It was evident that he knew what we were doing. When we went back to 5th floor, the CNA put him to bed. He was so tired; he wouldn't eat his lunch. I went on to work for about four hours, and came back by the nursing home. Ken was sitting at the dining room table for supper. He didn't eat very much, but he drank some liquids. He kept looking upward and sort of leaned forward and then asked, "Why?" and looked confused. The CNA put him to bed, and he was asleep almost as soon as his head was on the pillow.

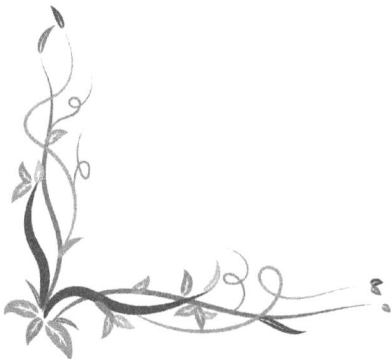

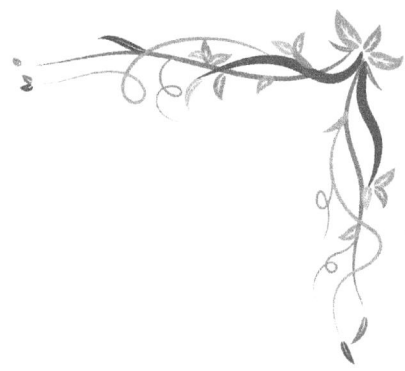

08/27/06

It was somewhere around this date that Chaplain Walker came to see Ken. Ken sat in his wheelchair facing me and Mr. Walker. Mr. Walker read some scripture and then sang. He asked if there was another song that I would like to hear. I suggested "It Is Well with My Soul." I held one of Ken's hands and Mr. Walker his other. When the song was finished, tears were running down Ken's cheeks. He raised both of his hands upward and waved them back and forth. I thought Mr. Walker was going to shout. He said, "Ken, you do know what we are talking and singing about." This was another way that God was reassuring me that all is well with his soul.

I've also been told that by this time Ken shouldn't have any idea who I am, nor aware of anything, but he does. Mr. Walker had said the same thing. Sometimes when I am feeding him, he doesn't seem to know me, but more often than not, he does.

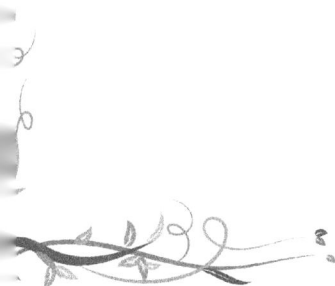

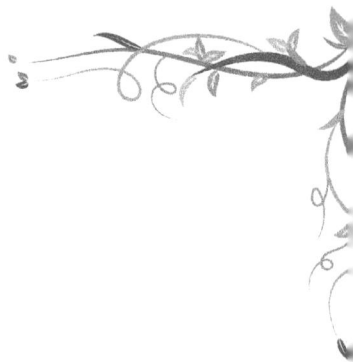

08/28/06

I had an endoscopy today. My friend Anne drove and looked after me. When we got home, she fixed me some soup which I ate, and then I went to bed. She has been a true friend.

The nurses agree with me that Ken needs a lot more sleep now. He can sleep after lunch, and within 1/2 hour after supper, his head is wobbling, and his eyes are going together.

09/03/06

I went to see Ken yesterday. He was about the same.

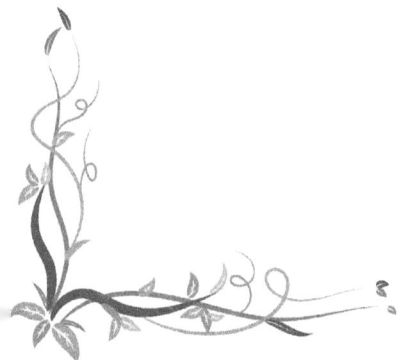

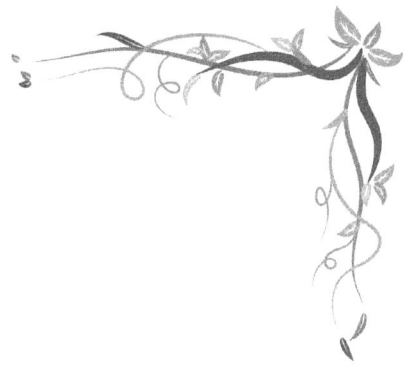

09/05/06

I went to see Ken after work. He had eaten supper, but he was watching the CNA getting the trays out of the carrier, as if he was starved. I hung his clothes up, put a light blanket over his arms, and pushed him outside. He is still nervous in an elevator. When we got outside, his whole demeanor seemed to change. He hummed a little, and made sounds as if he were sharing thoughts with someone, but not with me. He was observant of everything. When we got back inside, the CNA said she had really enjoyed the Gold City tape that she and Ken sang with during whirlpool bath. She said he would hum and laugh. I am so glad he has her. Also bathing in the whirlpool helps keep his fingernails clean.

09/06/06

The car light came on this morning about a mile down the expressway. It read to service engine soon. The car slowed down, and I was able to coast off the road. Trucks were flying by and each time, it seemed they would blow me off the road. Thank God for cell phones.

I called Nissan in W-S and then a tow truck. Then, I called Dwayne who works in same building that I do, to see if he would stop on his way in. He did, and then he brought me home. I'm to go by in the morning and pick it up. God always seems to be one step ahead.

I am so tired, but as am not sleeping well.

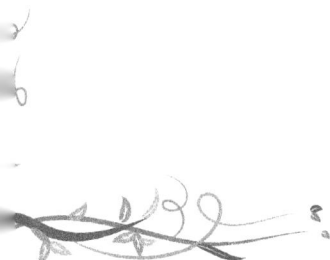

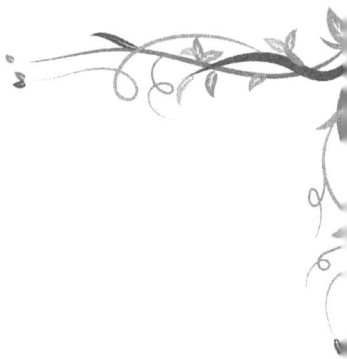

09/07/06

I didn't get my car until this afternoon. Dwayne has been so nice. He took me home yesterday, and let me ride in with him this morning, and took me by the Nissan place. It has been a long week. When I got the car, I went to see Ken. He still doesn't seem to be feeling good.

09/08/06

I had to take a day off work as FMLA today. My right foot was hurting really bad, and it seemed as if I couldn't focus on any one thing. I don't need to be driving when I'm this way. When I have the right medication, it helps with the pain, but there are times that I can't wear my shoes. I did go to Wal-Mart to get groceries late this afternoon. I didn't get home as soon as I had planned. I was completely worn out.

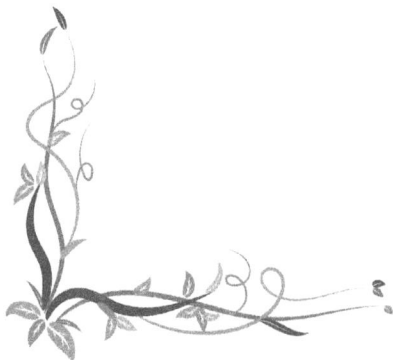

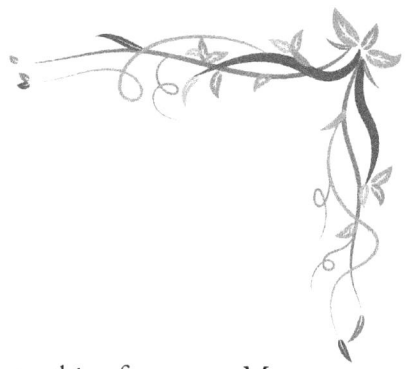

09/09/06

We gave Daddy a small 97th birthday party this afternoon. My niece, Laura helped with everything. Daddy was glad to see everyone, but just didn't feel like being up. He is so precious.

We got everything cleaned up about 5:00 p.m., and I went to see Ken. The weather was so nice, and I took him outside in his wheelchair for a while. When I first got off the elevator, he was watching the CNA taking out the food trays for the 2nd meal. The dining room is not large enough to feed all of the residents at the same time, plus some need more help than others. I asked her if Ken had eaten, and she said yes. I had to laugh 'cause he was watching every move she made as if he was starving to death. He eats everything on his plate, so I knew he wasn't that hungry.

He still doesn't like to ride on elevators. I usually put my arms around him and talk to calm him. He seemed to be happy to be outside. When I pushed his wheelchair out, he stopped, crossed his feet and just looked around. A man was loading his truck with a new demonstration bed for heavy people, and was having a difficult time. Ken was watching him very closely.

When I said let's go for a walk, he put his hand on the wheel, and steered it toward the man. I never cease to be amazed at the comprehension that Ken has. I pushed him up close enough for him to watch. The man was very nice. We talked about the Lord, and having patience. He had a 16 year old daughter whom I could tell that he was close to. We watched him until he finally got everything loaded, and then I pushed Ken back to the entrance. We went back to his room, and he was ready for bed. He seemed so sleepy. He seems to need more and more sleep.

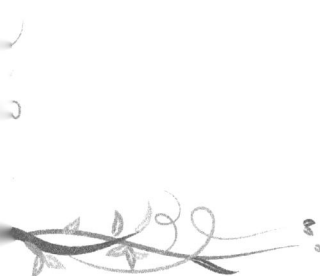

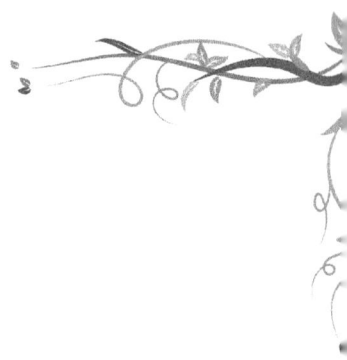

09/11/06

I went to see Ken after work today, and he was in the bed. They said he had been up, but about 5:00 p.m., he began to droop, so they put him to bed. He didn't appear to respond to me when I first saw him, but then he smiled at me. These moments come and go as quickly. He ate well, but strangled on the liquids. He refused to drink his juice, which he usually enjoys.

When I went in his room, the CNA was playing his tape by Jeff and Angel. It was so comforting. I then put on one that a friend had given me of Andy Griffith. By this time, Ken had eaten and was resting. All of a sudden, his chin began to tremble. His face changed and tears began running down his cheek, and just as quickly stopped. I sat there and cried with him. I was sitting in a chair beside his bed, and holding his hand. He kept a firm grip on it and squeezed it from time to time.

I stayed longer than usual. All of a sudden, Ken began to look around and then closed his eyes. He said, "Mama," twice. When I left, he was almost asleep. He seemed reAstless. I didn't want to leave, but knew I needed to.

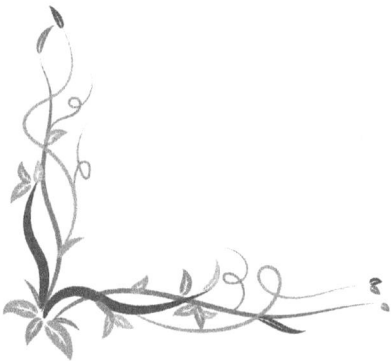

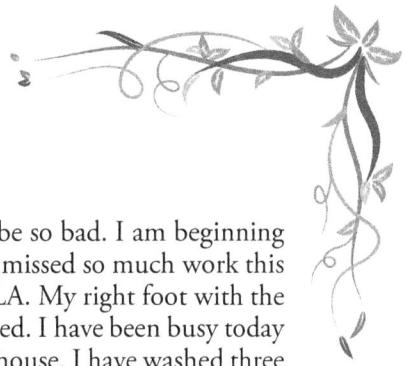

01/06/07

I do hope and pray that this next year will not be so bad. I am beginning to give out physically and emotionally again. I have missed so much work this past two months. I've used up almost all of my FMLA. My right foot with the osteoarthritis is extremely painful. It is swollen and red. I have been busy today trying to catch up on some things, like cleaning the house. I have washed three loads of clothes, one of which was Ken's. I plan to take to him when I visit him tomorrow.

A couple of months ago, I was out of work, and at home. The nursing home called and said Ken wasn't responding, and for me to be careful, but hurry. I got a ticket for speeding, and it seemed to take the patrolman forever to do his thing. This is the first ticket I have ever had. I explained to him what was happening, but he said it would be between me and the judge. (When I went to court, the judge was very nice, and said due to my good driving record, he was dismissing the charges. I could have hugged his neck.)

As it turned out, Hospice was at the nursing home when I got there, and had suctioned Ken, and had put him on oxygen for a while. I stayed with him that night, Thursday night, and Friday night. He coughed so hard and didn't know how to get the mucous out, and would swallow. It frightened him when this happened. He would groan so pitiful, and was so helpless. When he would have a coughing spell, he'd try to come out of the bed, and that made it easier for me to hold him up until he could relax. We kept his bed rolled up to almost a sitting position.

I didn't sleep for three nights. Gwen, my supervisor let me come home to sleep and go in to work late. I had called Susie, Ken's sister, and she and his brother Roger came to stay with him some on Friday. She came Thursday, and so did Chaplain Walker, who was so nice. He stayed for a while and had prayer before he left. Gerald, our pastor, and Tim, one of the deacons, came on Wednesday night. Ken knew Gerald. He laughed, and reached out his hand for a handshake. It was so good to see them, and it was a comfort to me.

There are times it seems that Ken is aware of my presence, but just as quickly, he's back in his world.

A couple of days ago, Ken was watching something that I couldn't see, and all of a sudden he brought both of his hands together up beside his shoulder. Someone not familiar with him would have thought he was going to hit them, but I knew, in his mind, he was hitting a baseball. Awesome to watch these glimpses of another place, another time.

Another night, we were sitting in the dining room facing the windows. The way the light was shining, we could see ourselves in them. Ken kept looking, and would move a little. All of a sudden, he said really loud, "Strike." He continued concentrating, and then he said, "Ball!" I couldn't help but wonder who he was seeing, as he umpired a ball game.

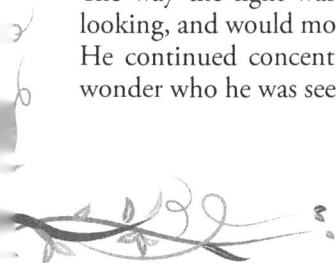

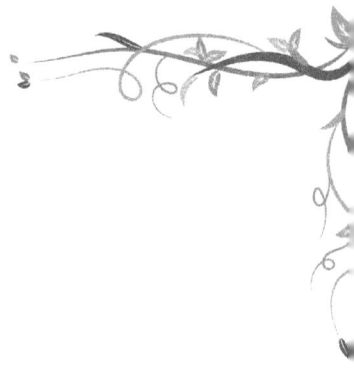

01/14/07

I am so tired that I'm weak as a noodle that's been overcooked. I went by to see Ken after work. I hung his clean clothes up, and put his PJ's in his allotted space.

The CNA had already fed him, showered him, and put him to bed. She said he was whipped when they finished. He sort of ignored me when I walked in the room.

I turned the tape recorder on of "Gold City." When Ken heard the music and singing, his face lit up. He looked at me and laughed. I massaged his head, and he tried to talk to me. Then he appeared to be somewhere else, and all of a sudden he said what sounded like "Where's the batter?" When I responded by asking, "Are you umpiring a ball game?" he looked at me and grinned.

The staff had pizza for supper, and it smelled so good. Ken's CNA asked me if I would like a slice and I told him not to throw any away, but wait until everyone else had eaten. If there was any left, then I'd eat a slice. The next thing I knew, he walked in with a big slice that he had microwaved for me. It was so good.

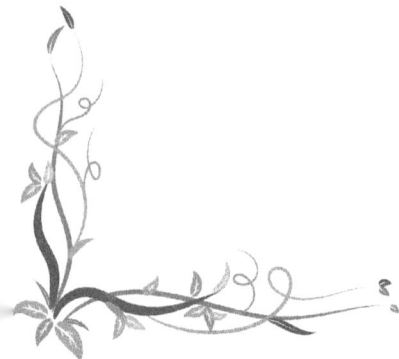

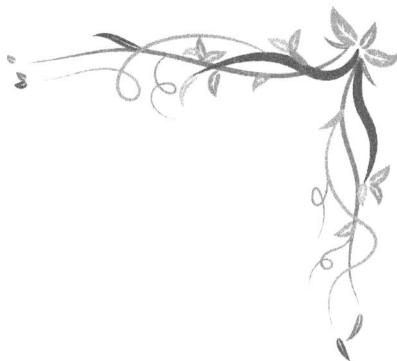

01/15/07 Monday 10:37 pm

I am so tired and so sleepy. Today was my first day back to work since last Tuesday. I had originally missed quite a few days with bronchitis, and before it completely cleared up, osteoarthritis was in my right knee and right foot. I have never seen my foot this large, nor my knee. The swelling is beginning to go down, but my foot and knee still hurt.

I haven't been to see Daddy in four weeks. I really miss him. I did get to go see Ken this evening. I shaved him, and washed his face real good. Then, I cut and cleaned his toenails, and fingernails. In his own way, he let me know that he wished I would go somewhere else, and leave him alone.

His CNA said that she turned on his tape and as she turned around, there were big tears falling down his cheek. No one can tell me that he doesn't know what is happening to him. So tough to watch him this way, and I know even tougher for him, as he can't get us to understand him. When I understand something he has mumbled or understood an action, he gets so excited and just laughs.

Oh, well, time to get clothes out of the dryer, and go to bed!

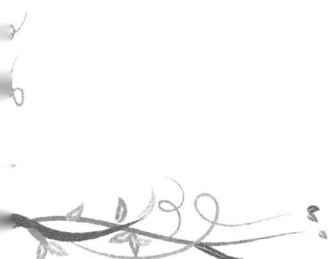

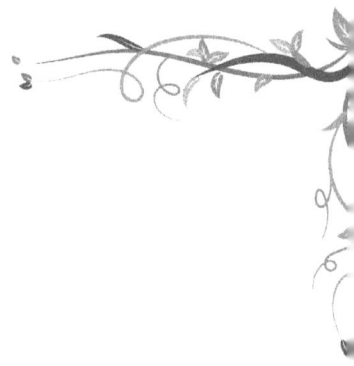

01/29/07

I have been missing so much work, and payments are behind on everything. I applied for assistance at work for my behind house payment. I went to see a counselor at Hospice today. She was very supportive, and wants me to bring some of my poems, and the journal on Ken next week. She named the things that I have been dealing with for such a long a time, and said she is amazed that I haven't folded before now. She suggested that I try again to follow Dr. Beaver's advice, and not go every day to see Ken. She agrees with me that I may need some type of medication change, and we will see if we can change my schedule.

I went to see Ken, and he was already in bed. His eyes sort of smiled when he saw me. He said something that I couldn't understand. I patted him on the cheek, and his mouth opened like a little bird. I went down the hall and got some thickening water from the nurse. Ken drank all of it. He put his hands behind his head, and closed his eyes as if going to sleep. I gathered his dirty clothes and left.

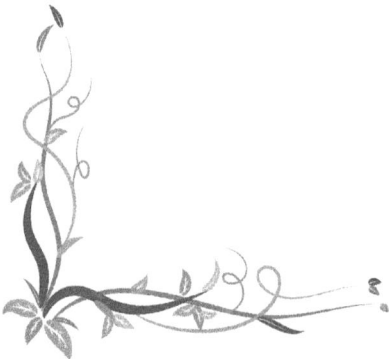

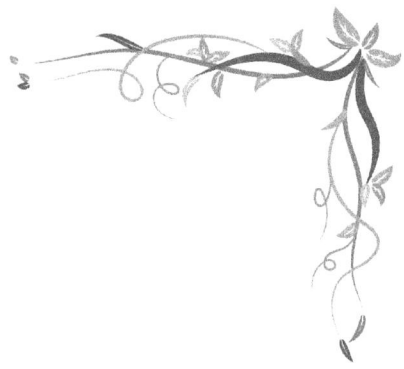

04/17/07

My right elbow has been swollen, and I can't move it as I should. I called and left a message that I wouldn't be in to work again. This bothers me. I have no energy, and am not alert enough to be driving. I had to gather information for Medicaid. I always get very nervous when they ask for something.

My friend, Anne, called and asked me to meet her for supper. I went, but only got a slice of cake. It's a good feeling to have a friend who wants to be with me. I still feel so lonely. When I first began going to a restaurant by myself, I would take a book with me. After placing my order, I could bury my head in the pages, and pretend that I wasn't alone.

04/18/07

My arm is still hurting. My life is so unsettled. I received a call from Medicaid, and I felt much better after talking with them. I went in to work.

I came home, was so tired, and sleepy, but couldn't sleep. I feel and know that I'm not very productive at work. There are some co-workers who make snide remarks about me, but they haven't walked in my shoes. I pray they never have to deal with a situation such as this.

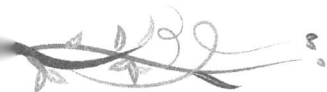

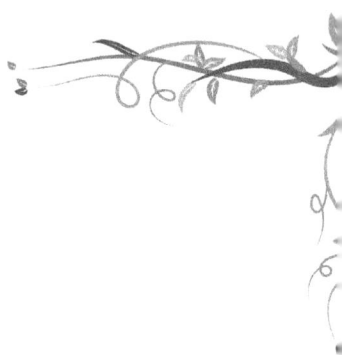

04/19/07

After work, I went to see Ken, who looked at me with those big baby blues, and he just laughed. He held my hand, and didn't want to let go. He tried to talk to me. I asked if he was hungry, and he said, "Yeah." When the CNA brought him his snack, he opened his mouth before she got to him. When she began talking to me, he grunted 'cause she wasn't feeding him fast enough. He's done me that way before. He later slowly moved his hand toward me, and I asked if he wanted a hug, and he said, "Yeah." When I hugged him, and lay my head next to his, and kissed his cheek, he said, "Ummmm." It's so sad, and I feel so helpless. So much is out of my control, and there is only so much I can do.

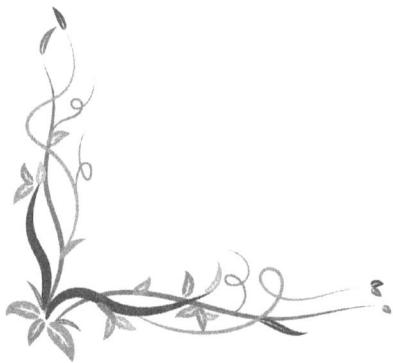

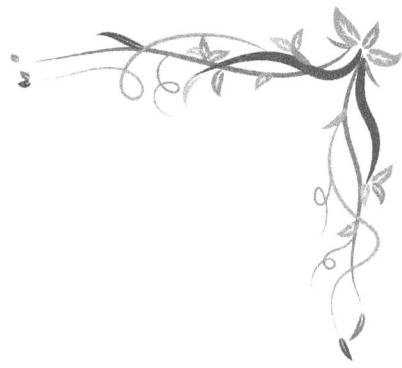

04/20/07

I went to Human Resources to get my new ID tag. After I finally found a parking space, I realized that I didn't have enough money, so I had to leave and go to the bank. When I got to HR I was told the cost would be taken out by payroll deduction. I went to work, but didn't work as long as I had planned, as I had finished what had been given to me.

I went to see Ken, who seemed happy to see me. I fed him supper, and then we went outside. He seems to come alive when he's outside. When I asked if he wanted to go outside, he became so excited. Later, I went out to eat with my friend, Kay, which was good for me. Everyone needs a friend like Kay.

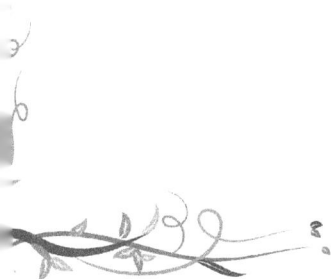

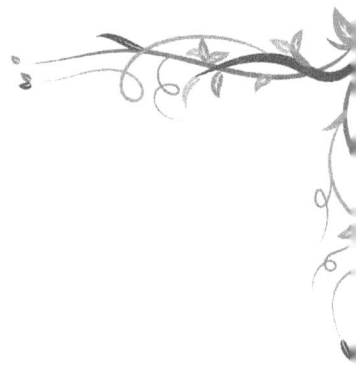

04/21/07

I needed to mow the yard. It was beginning to look like a jungle. A friend called, and asked me to go with our church group to the Barn Theater. They assured me that my ticket was already paid. I had such a wonderful time, the food was so delicious, the music was lovely and I laughed so much! One of the performers, Grace, was a beautiful young lady from our church. I thought of Ken, especially when a song was sung that he liked, and I cried. But, I survived!

I also worked in the yard some today. I never know when the osteoarthritis is going to knock me off my feet, and am so thankful when I can accomplish something worthwhile.

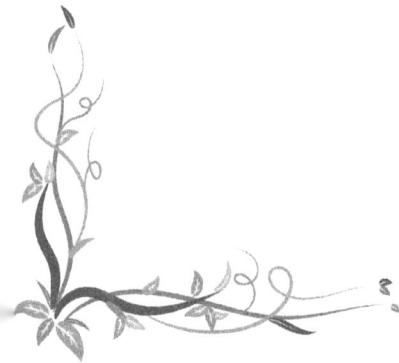

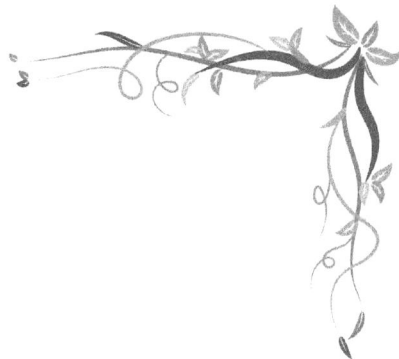

04/22/07

I didn't sleep much last night. I ate breakfast, and attended church with my brother. I enjoy listening and watching him pick his guitar. I thoroughly enjoyed myself.

I went to see Daddy after church. I pushed Daddy outside in the fresh air. I always enjoy spending time with him. I try to keep his hair trimmed, and feel it a privilege to do this.

After visiting with Daddy, I went to see Ken and cut his hair. When Lewana's schedule doesn't allow her to do the honors, I try. He doesn't always sit still, and I don't always do a good job. I'll tell Ken that we're going to have to tell Polly to do better next time, and he'll laugh.

We went outside for a while, and when we went back in, I fed him his snack. I had to laugh at him. I was shaving him, and when he was ready for me to leave him alone, he took hold of my arm, and wouldn't let go. I've learned to appreciate the humor in small things in order to survive.

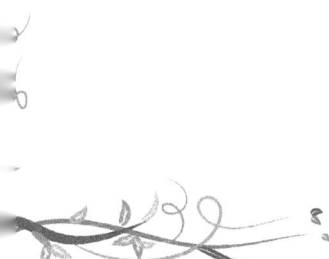

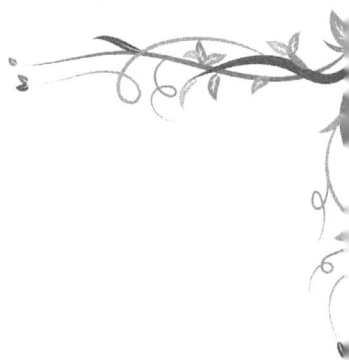

04/23/07

I didn't sleep very well last night, and did not have a good day at work. I had an appointment with Otolaryngology this morning, and got my new hearing aids.

I went to see my counselor this afternoon. It's always good to talk with her. She is so encouraging, and after a day like I had, I needed it. I came home, and mowed part of the yard. There's something about mowing, and being outside that helps clear the cobwebs.

04/25/07

I had a busy day at work. It had been a beautiful day outside. I wanted to take Ken out, but by the time I got there, it was too late. I'm not sure if he actually recognized me, but he was doing a lot of reaching upward and looking around at the ceiling. One time he said "Bye," but he wasn't talking to me. I was so tired when I got home.

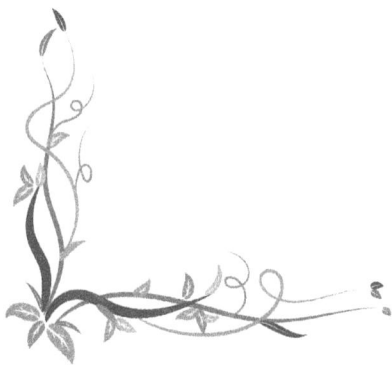

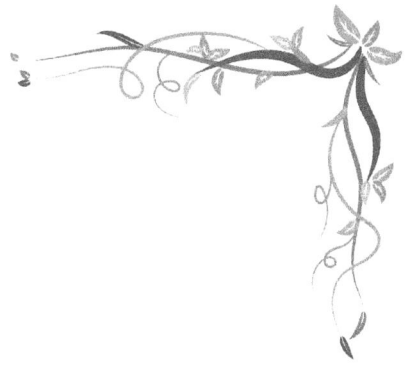

04/26/07

It was so hard to get up this morning. I ate breakfast, and took a shower. My body and mind is so tired. I did recycling at work, and was on my feet for 2 ½ hours. They were so swollen when I got home.

I put turf builder on the lawn. It was good to be outside, and good to be home. I put Ken's clothes in to wash, will put in the dryer before I go to bed, and fold them in the morning. I wore my hearing aids today and yesterday. It will take a while to adjust to them.

I received a call about my loan. I had already been to the bank this morning, and didn't have enough to get any cash. Family and friends have helped me before, and I'm not going to ask them again. I have found that God always comes through.

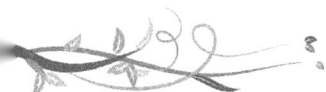

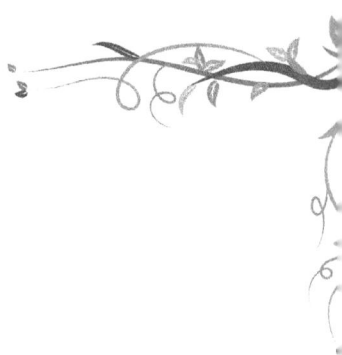

04/27/07

I didn't sleep much last night, and have no energy. I did get some happy news. I have a new great-great niece named Cassie Jade.

I went to Wal-Mart to get groceries. When I tried to pay for them, the machine wouldn't take my Wal-Mart card. I was so embarrassed. I'm back home, no groceries, and wonder what tomorrow holds. Right now I feel hopeless, and helpless. I need to remember that God will never leave me nor forsake me.

04/28/07

I didn't sleep any last night, but I've had a busy day. I guess I was going on nervous energy. I washed clothes, took trash to the dump, went to the post office, and when I came home, I tried to crank the lawnmower. When I couldn't do that, I did some weed eating until the power gave out. I had to recharge it. I cleaned up the car port, ate and rested in between chores. Every joint and muscle is aching. My hot shower sure did feel good.

During this difficult time, I was trying to visit to my dad in the hospital. I also would go by to see Ken, and took his clothes home with me to wash. As I tried to continue with normal responsibilities, I lost track of time, days, etc.

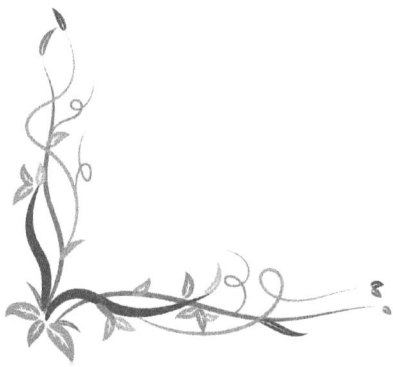

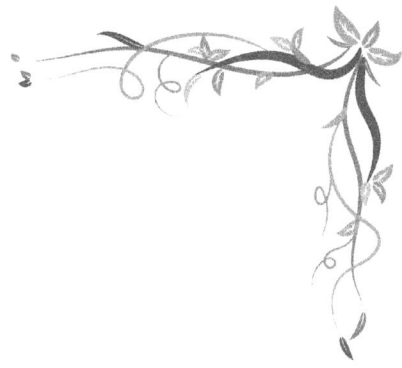

05/15/07 Tuesday

I left work around 2:00 p.m., and was about halfway home, and my brother called to let me know that the nursing home was sending Daddy to the hospital. I went home as he had planned to ride with me. He then called and said he would ride with our niece, Laura. I got to the Emergency Room and Daddy knew me. He also knew Russell and Laura. They had already put in IV's and done a chest x-ray. He was breathing so hard, and was thirsty. I was allowed to give him some ice chips which helped. He had double pneumonia. I stayed with him that night. The antibiotic wasn't helping, and he was fighting for every breath he was getting. I'd stay with him until around 2:00 a.m., go home to rest, and go back.

I had to stay off of my feet, because of gout for a couple of days. But, I did stay all night with him before he was moved to the Hospice House. He died there on *May 26, 2007*, which was a memorial day weekend. The night before he was moved, he knew me and my brother, and the grand-children who were there, but had difficulty saying I LOVE YOU. He would try so hard. Of course, it was hurtful for us to see him like this. Such a precious person who loved everyone he knew, and was such a faithful child of God.

Russell and I, with Laura's help took care of finalizing funeral arrangements. I had already called to let Jeff and Angel know that it was just a matter of time, and wanted them to sing "Going Home" as he was being taken out of the church. Gerald, Brent and Joan sang the two songs that Daddy had chosen years ago, and Jeanette played piano. They were "The Old Rugged Cross" and" In the Sweet By and By."

The osteoarthritis was so bad by this time, that I wasn't able to attend his funeral. My friend, Anne stayed with me so I wouldn't be alone. *Anne, a one of a kind friend has since gone to heaven.*

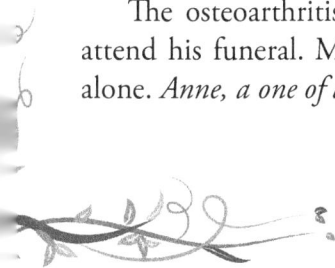

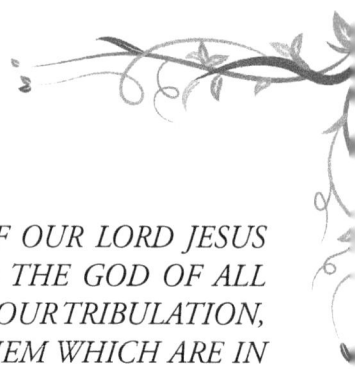

II CORINTHIANS 1: 3,4

BLESSED BE GOD, EVEN THE FATHER OF OUR LORD JESUS CHRIST, THE FATHER OF MERCIES, AND THE GOD OF ALL COMFORT; WHO COMFORTETH US IN ALL OUR TRIBULATION, THAT WE MAY BE ABLE TO COMFORT THEM WHICH ARE IN ANY TROUBLE, THE COMFORT WHEREWITH WE OURSELVES ARE COMFORTED OF GOD.

HEBREWS 11::1

NOW FAITH IS THE SUBSTANCE OF THINGS HOPED FOR, THE EVIDENCE OF THINGS NOT SEEN.

JOHN 3:16

FOR GOD SO LOVED THE WORLD, THAT HE GAVE HIS ONLY BEGOTTEN SON, THAT WHOSOEVER BELIEVETH IN HIM SHOULD NOT PERISH, BUT HAVE EVERLASTING LIFE.

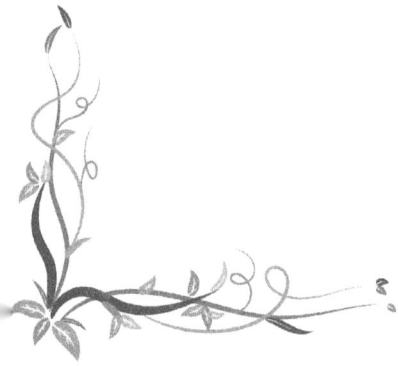

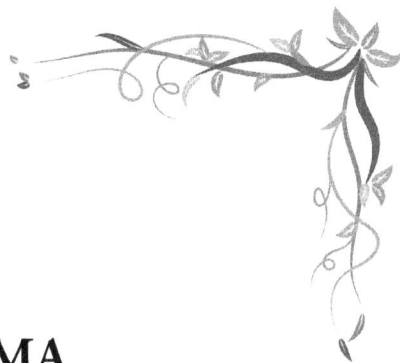

DADDY & MAMA

Mama reached out her hand to Daddy.
Without hesitation
he reached out and took her hand.
The look on their faces, and the love in their eyes
had come from years of sharing
whatever life sent their way.
They could be seen holding hands
as fate dealt such a bitter blow.
It seemed they could hardly stand beneath
the weight of the load.
They could hold on a little longer
as they drew strength from each other
and from the Lord whom they both loved.
As the ebbing tide slowly washed away the sands of time,
they still held each other's hand
as their time on earth together
step by step came to an end…
Now God has reunited Daddy and Mama in Heaven
where once again they
hold each other's hand.

May 24, 2007

(My Mama passed away in March, 1987, and my Daddy in May,
2007. My sister Jacqueline, who was forty-nine, was killed in a car wreck
09/85, and my brother's daughter Renee' who was seventeen, was killed
in a car wreck two weeks later 10/85. I wrote this poem originally in
1995, and that was 10 years after my Mama died, but put a new ending
for Daddy's funeral.)

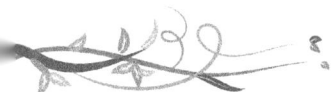

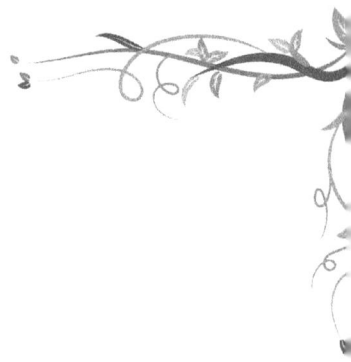

06/05/07 Tuesday

Time has a way of slipping by you like a ship in the night, and you can't help but wonder, "What have I missed?" I have noticed that Ken is not laughing, nor smiling as much as he did. He sleeps a lot more, but I have also noticed that he is often restless.

He has a way like a ritual that he has to go thru, to get to sleep. He doesn't do this all the time, but quite often. He keeps pulling on the sheets and works his arms back and forth. I have tried to accommodate him, but have realized that I need to leave him alone, and let him do his thing. He keeps pulling on the sheets until he gets them over his head and his hands around and under his head. Then he begins to relax.

Ken has had a good relationship with Chaplain Craig Walker, and Katie, the music therapist. One of his sisters' sings to him and he tries to move his mouth as if trying to sing, and sometimes you can hear something that sounds like humming.

Before I leave after a visit, I try to remember to leave one of his tapes playing. There seems to be a peaceful look on his face. He is still sitting up in bed, and reaching upward, looking around, and having conversations that no one else is included in. I feel this is his time that the angels in Heaven are showing him things yet to come, and to let him know that he's not alone.

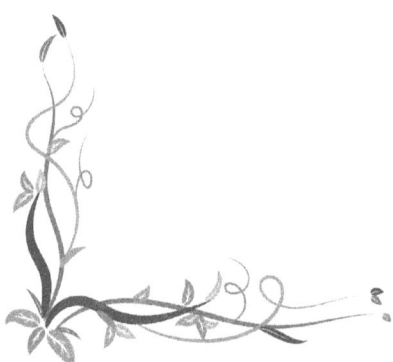

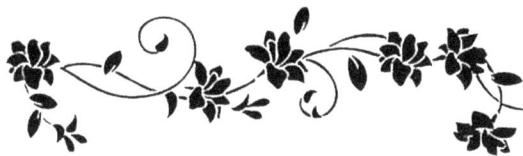

UNTIL THEN

My heart is full of pain and despair.
It seems at times the burden is too hard to bear.
As I sit by your bedside holding your hand,
I can't help but wonder how much of this you understand.
Music softly plays as you try to hum the song.
The words to "I'll fly away" is heard so clearly,
As your face lights up and you say, "Yeah."
You reach up toward Heaven, but God lets
You know that it's not yet time,
And tells you that until then,
"I'll keep your hand in Mine."

06/15/07

The last few times that I have been to see Ken, he hasn't seemed to recognize me. He has held my hand. I sang Happy Birthday to him, and it looked like there were tears in his eyes. He turned 62 on June 04, 2007.

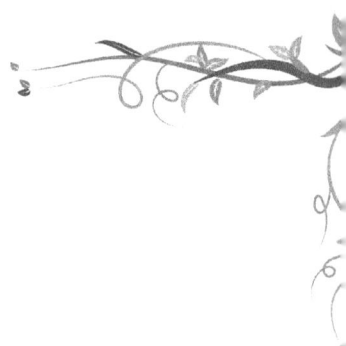

I haven't been working very much. I do like the option of going in later, but it seems that I am still so tired. I talked to Dr. Beavers about retirement on disability, and he said I would definitely qualify. I talked with my work disability person. She is so nice. Of course, this is a long drawn out case of who is going to let me know something and when.

I was told to go to a psychiatrist in order to have my ducks in a row. It seems they must have been swimming in someone else's pond. No one is letting me know anything. I'm very confused and there is so much going on.

****

June 17, 2007

Laura, my niece came to get me to ride with her to Winston Salum, and then to her house for Father's Day supper with her family. I had a great time. I enjoy spending time with her, and her family. I did alright until her father-in-law returned thanks for our food. In my mind I was hearing Daddy.

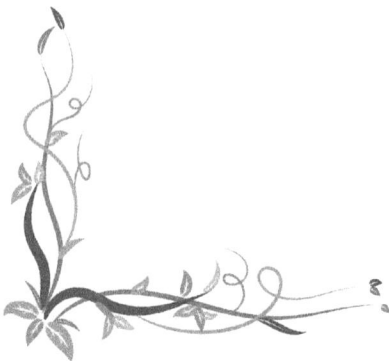

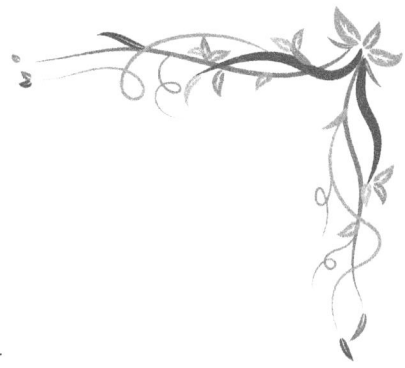

June 20, 2007 Wed

I have missed my Dad so much. We were so blessed to have his hugs and I love you's. His birthday would have been in September 13, 2007. We lost almost 98 years of wisdom, but he gained Heaven.

I went back to my doctor and was put on Prednisone yesterday, and I can tell it has helped me. My foot is still swollen and painful, but not nearly as bad.

I went to see Ken this afternoon, and he was already in bed. His eyes recognized me, and he tried to say something to me. I bent over to hug him, and he was making the hugging sound before I hugged him. That told me that he was aware. His eyes followed me around the room, and he seemed to be thirsty. I went to get him some thickening and a little ice to mix with his grape drink that I keep for him. He swallowed it, and opened his mouth for more. He then said, "I want it," and he drank about 7 oz for me. He laughed some during this, and would say something that wasn't understandable. *Times like this are so difficult.*

I put on the tape by Jeff and Angel that he enjoys, and he tried to sing with them. He was moving his toes in time with the music, and then I noticed his fingers. He seemed to be strumming and cording his guitar.

I came home, and put his clothes in the washer. Got to go put in dryer, and get ready for bed.

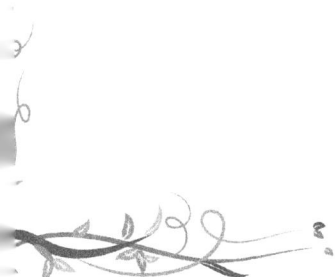

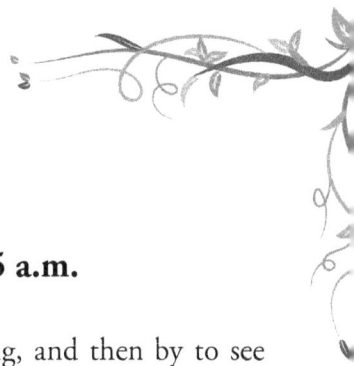

June 23, 2007 Friday 12:45 a.m.

I went for my physical therapy this morning, and then by to see Ken. He was in the dining room waiting for his tray. Some of the others had theirs, and he kept looking at theirs, and looked at me so pitiful. He couldn't understand why he didn't have his yet.

I talked to him, and gave him a hug. He didn't say anything, but had a smile on his face. His tray was put on the table, and I fed him. He didn't eat all of his food, closed his mouth, and turned his head. He did drink his milk, and ½ of his water. I still can tell a difference in his swallowing. No one else seems to think it's different.

Ken's doctor was making his rounds, and I talked with him about the CNA. changing his Depends the last two times I was there. They used several wet-wipes. Ken's doctor said that he would order an enema every 3rd day. He made the comment that his bowels were probably beginning to stop. He stated what I had felt. I told him that I had asked the nurses about it, but they didn't seem to be concerned. He also agreed with me, that Ken needs to have more bed rest than in the past. I told him that the CNA's were not consistent in putting him to bed.

I went to work, came home and mowed part of the yard. Jean had left me some fresh squash, new potatoes, and zucchini. I fried some squash, and ate about 9:00 p.m., took my shower, and I am ready for bed.

Lewana called this morning, and we met at K & W for lunch. It was so nice just being with her. We then went to see Ken. He was in bed, but not asleep. The CNA put him in his wheelchair, and Lewana cut his hair. He stayed so still, and when she was ready to cut on his lower left side, I held his head so she could get to it. He is beginning to lean more and more to his left.

We cleaned everything up, washed his hair, and put a clean shirt on him. Then, we took him outside. It was hot, so we sat in the shade. A couple of young men appeared to be looking under the hood of a car. Ken wasn't missing any of that. Lewana went back inside, and brought him some thickened grape drink. He drank all of it.

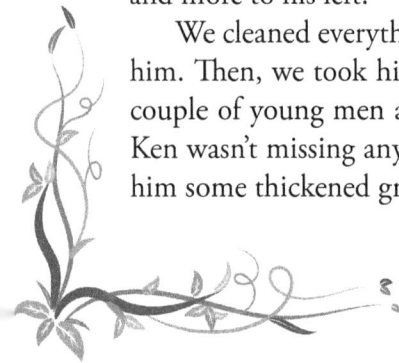

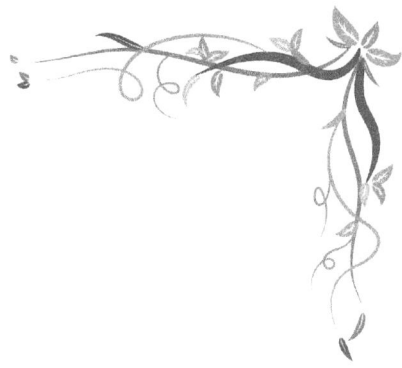

07/01/07 Sunday 10:30 pm

My friend Anne treated me for lunch. We didn't have to hurry, and went to see Ken afterwards. We got to the nursing home approximately 4:10 p.m. When we walked into his room, he was in his wheelchair, slumped over his lap-buddy, head hanging down, and his hands were on the floor. He was propping himself up with his right hand. His hand and arm was red midway to his elbow. I immediately went to get his nurse. I kept talking to Ken, and trying to pull him up, but couldn't.

Alex and another nurse came and had to work with him, before finally getting him in the bed. He was confused and frightened. When he saw me, he smiled so pitifully, and reached his hand to me. I took hold of it, and kept trying to reassure him that he was alright, even though I knew he wasn't.

I told his nurse that I was very upset, and I would be making a call tomorrow to get to the bottom of this. He told me the two CNA's names who had Ken this morning. They took him to his room at approximately 1:00 pm. He thought they were putting Ken to bed, but didn't actually see them. He said they usually get him up for his snack. He didn't know how long he had been up, but said they have their snack around 2:00 p.m. So in that case, he had been sitting in his wheelchair for two hours, or four hours, and no one had checked on him.

Even after being put to bed, Ken couldn't seem to relax. He was jerking all over, the way he would while having a seizure. He kept holding to my hand. I washed his face, which hadn't been shaved.

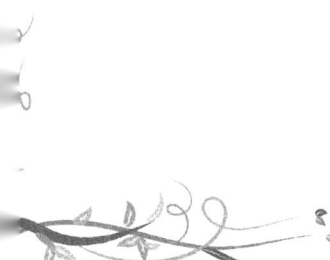

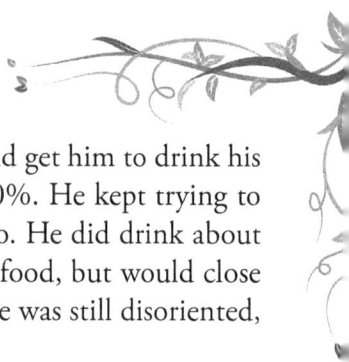

When his supper came, I tried to feed him and get him to drink his liquids. He only ate and drank approximately 20%. He kept trying to open his mouth, but was having trouble doing so. He did drink about all of his milk, and tea. He ate a few bites of his food, but would close his mouth, and act as if he didn't want it. Also, he was still disoriented, kept jerking, and moving his feet and legs.

The CNA came in and pulled him up in bed, but he kept turning to his left side. The CNA and the nurse changed him, and then the nurse gave him his medicine. (They are both so kind and compassionate with Ken). He took a while, and did the same thing that I had done, by rubbing on his neck to get him to swallow. I had complained about this for some time, but reaction from staff and the therapist was nonchalant, and didn't see any difference.

There is now a new therapist who has told them to massage his neck muscles to get him to swallow, per his nurse. No one has mentioned this to me. They then put on his pajamas, and straightened him in bed. He appeared to be more comfortable, and so sleepy. I felt that he would go to sleep when we left. I called back about 9:30 p.m., and his nurse said he drank 1/2 of his liquid when he gave him his medicine, but had not slept. The sad thing is if there is no one with him, and if he has another seizure, it isn't recorded. This type of trauma can trigger one. The only thing that I didn't notice was his eyes rolling back. This just wore him out.

It's 11:00 p.m. and I'm ready for bed. I am so tired. I pray for strength needed to deal with things tomorrow. I have physical therapy in the morning. The repairman is supposed to work on the dryer again (4th).

I have an appointment with Dr. Graham Thursday, to find out results of my ultrasound, and he will do more blood work. It has been really hard to stay off meats for 2 weeks. I finally gave in Friday and got me a chicken breast and cream potatoes. It was so good.

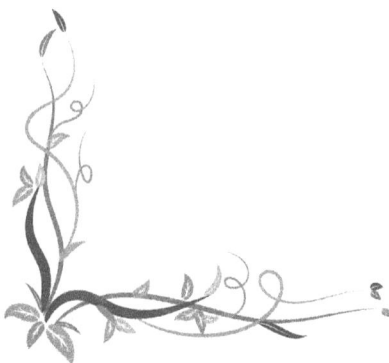

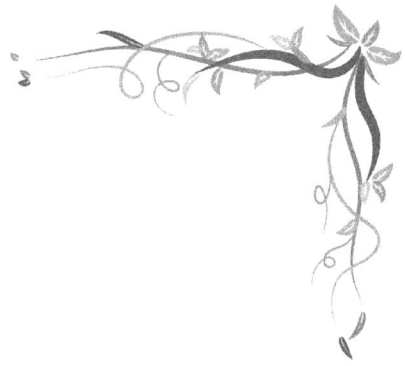

07/02/07 Monday

I called the nursing home this morning, after physical therapy, to see when we could discuss the problems of yesterday. She said to come on to her office. I had my notes, and covered everything. I let her know how furious I was, how helpless Ken was, how disoriented and frightened he was. I gave her the two CNA's names and the nurse's. She said she would talk with them to get to the bottom of what happened, and will let me know. She was appalled that he had been found that way. She agreed with me that it was likely that he could have a seizure as result of the trauma. We discussed the amount of time that he was left alone and no one checking on him.

After speaking with the nurse, I went up to check on him. He was in his wheelchair close to the nurses' station with his feet stretched out, and his head hanging backward. I went back and asked the nurse to go with me. When we got off the elevator, he was trying to hold his head up, and his eyes were like saucers and he was confused. He was also leaning over his lap-buddy. He just could not hold himself up. She immediately told the CNA to put him to bed. This was approximately 11:00 a.m. He went to sleep almost as soon as they laid him down.

I went on to work, and then back to check on Ken. I got there around 7:00 p.m. He was in the bed with his PJ'S on. The bed was rolled up at the head, and Ken's head was already moving to his left. He doesn't stay straight anymore.

The CNA said he ate a good supper, but did not drink much liquid. His nurse mixed thickener with some grape drink, and I gave Ken about three tiny tastes of it. He tried to lick it off his mouth, but some ran down the side.

The next thing I knew he was coming straight up in bed, trying to cough, and he was fighting to breathe. It was more like getting choked than being strangled. He looked at me so pitiful, as if he couldn't understand why I couldn't do anything. It scared him and me. I helped hold him up, until he began to relax and lay back. He had such a bad

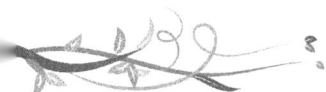

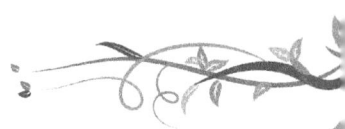

spell that I hollered for his nurse. I was working with Ken trying to help him get his breath back. I finally ran to the door and hollered for his nurse several times. I thought I heard someone say they'd be there in a minute. I didn't see the emergency button to push, even though it was probably there.

I waited an hour, and still no one came. In the meantime, Ken was so restless. He would look as if he was going to sleep, and then would have a coughing spell. I took hold of his hand, and he was waving both his arms up over his head, the same way he did when Chaplain Walker sang "It Is Well with My Soul."

Ken kept playing with his sheet. I put both of his hands under his head after watching him try, and his right arm kept sliding back down. This is the way he usually goes to sleep. He will cover his head with the sheet and put both hands under his head. I lay the sheet across the top of his head, and side of his face. Within almost no time, he relaxed and went to sleep. I didn't leave until 9:30 p.m.

Ken's nurse came to check on him. He told me that he was having supper when I called for him. I told him that Ken could have died in my arms, and no one would have cared. Not a soul came to see what was happening. I will have to talk with someone tomorrow. I was uneasy leaving him tonight.

On my way home, I called Anne, and she said to come by and eat chicken pie and she had Jell-O and whipped cream. It tasted so good. I got home at 11:00 p.m. I put in some clothes to dry. The repairman came today. Still not sure the dryer is fixed.

It is now 2:00 a.m., and I'm going to bed. I am exhausted, but wanted to get this documented. I called and left a message for Gwen that I would be late for work tomorrow. I plan to go by the nursing home first thing in the morning.

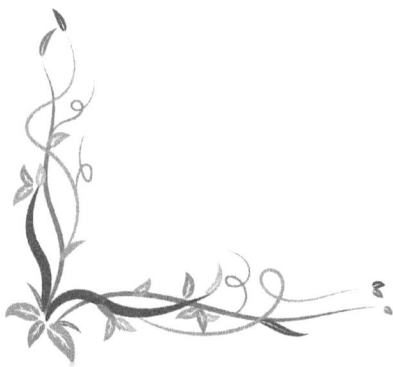

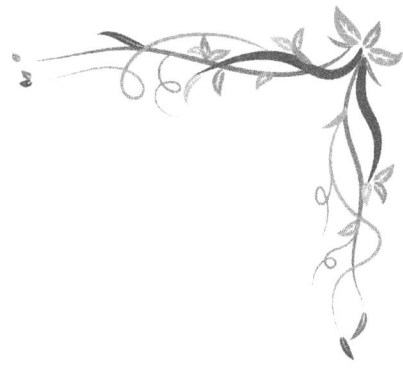

07/03/07 Tuesday

I called and spoke with the director of nursing about last night's events. We also discussed again the occupational therapy evaluating him, and speech therapy, because of the swallowing and choking. She still couldn't tell me anything in reference to Sunday's episode. She questioned me again as to how I came up with the CNA's names. She did talk with the nurse, and he told her he didn't see Ken put to bed. If I understood correctly, he gave her the CNA's name. Tonight I went back by after work, and Ken is still not doing good; very restless.

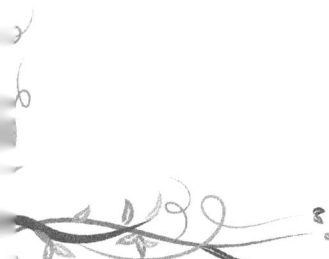

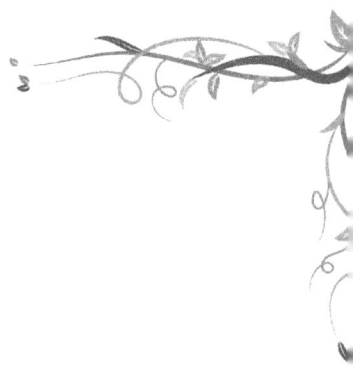

07/04/07 Wednesday

Didn't go see Ken today. I mowed the yard, and felt that I need to take care of Polly, as Dr. Beaver keeps telling me. Very beautiful day.

07/05/07 Thursday

I went by to check on Ken on my way in to work. When I went by to check on Ken after work, his head had rolled off his pillow. It was up against the bumper pad with his face under the bumper pad. The head of the bed is left up more now because of the strangling. I went down the hall and got the agency nurse.

I asked her to come with me, so I could show her how I had found him. I asked her to have him checked more often, and that he needed some type of cushion between his pillow and the pads. She said she will pass the word along. I'm uneasy about leaving him.

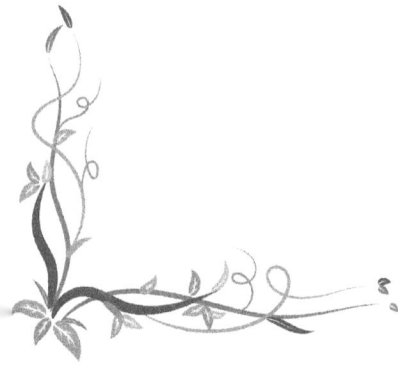

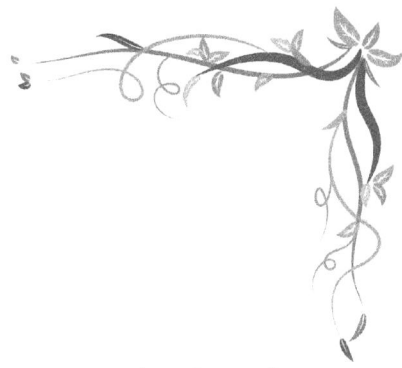

07/06/07 Friday

I had called yesterday, and again today, for occupational and speech therapy to call me, and neither returned my call. I finally spoke with the therapist who had requested that a Brody chair be put in Ken's room.

She said that she will check with both therapies, and will tell nurses and staff that Ken is to wear a hospital gown at night now. I really feel he needs to wear it all of the time. I plan to go tomorrow and will see what I feel at that time. She will also see that paperwork is taken care of for Hospice to be reinstated per my request.

The nurse on duty tonight, was so patient with me and Ken, trying to make him comfortable. He just could not be still. He'd slide his feet up and down, and then bring his knees up to his stomach, and would groan so helplessly. I feel he is hurting somewhere, but can't tell us. The nurse checked his bladder, and said no distention, no bowel blockage, heart rate good. I felt so sorry for him.

Ken just wore himself out trying to get comfortable enough to sleep. She gave him his Ativan about 8:00 pm, and was going to give him Darvacet ground up in applesauce, but by the time she got around to him, he had finally relaxed enough to go to sleep.

Prior to that his eyes were closed, but he wasn't resting. He'd holler and try to come up out of the bed. He did a lot of looking around tonight, and seeing things that I couldn't.

The third shift nurse was there when I left, and she said she will call me if anything changes. The 2nd shift nurse got the portable suction machine and placed beside Ken's bed to have ready. He has really plummeted the last two weeks. It's 3:00 a.m. Got to go to bed.

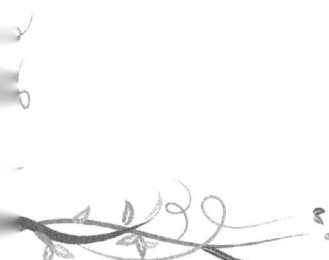

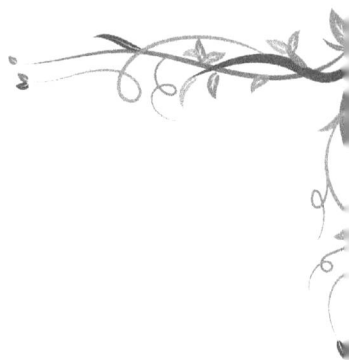

07/07/07 Saturday

I have kept rather busy today doing basic housecleaning that I don't always get to do. I had hoped to bake zucchini bread, but ran out of time. I could have stayed home. After I took my shower, I called Anne to see if she would go with me to church, so I could practice on the organ and piano. My piano is so out of tune, it warbles. We were there over two hours, and I had such a relaxing time. It was just what the doctor ordered.

I called to check on Ken, and the nurse said he is not eating very much, and would hold food in his mouth without swallowing it. She said he did the same with his thickened liquids and it would run down the corner of his face. I told her that I plan to come down tomorrow, if I can walk. My feet are pretty swollen tonight and very painful. I can't have any more medication for pain in my feet tonight.

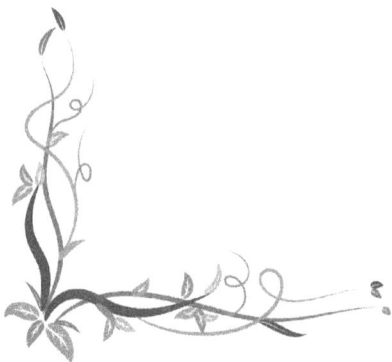

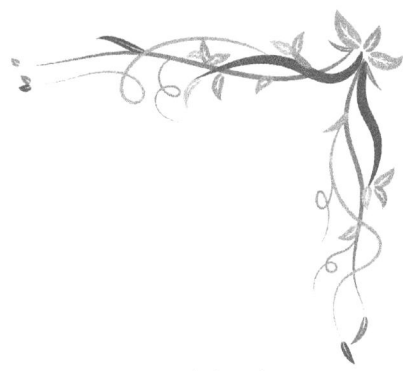

07/08/07 Sunday

Gerald called and said he had just left from visiting Ken, and that he could tell that he is much weaker. I got there about 6:00 p.m. and the CNA. said he only ate and drank about 50%. I question that, but didn't say anything. The nurse said he is having such a time getting choked. She said, "When food or liquid is put in his mouth, the muscles don't connect telling him to swallow." He was so pathetic.

One of the times he started choking, he looked at me and saw me crying, and his eyes told me he knew. At different times as I held his hand, he would weakly squeeze it. I finally asked the nurse if anyone had talked with the doctor. She immediately left a message for him to call. When the doctor returned her call, she told him what she had observed, and my questions of what to do at this point, to keep him comfortable, etc.

As of in the morning, his Ativan is to be increased to four times a day, as needed for pain or agitation. He is also to be given something to dry up the mucous. He also asked the nurse to contact Hospice and she faxed them the request. They will get in touch with me in the morning and reevaluate him. Kim from Hospice wanted to talk with me. When I told her that we were already on file, she said that she remembered our name.

The doctor also asked to speak with me, and told me how sorry he was, but that we both knew this time was coming. He said even though we know this, nothing can really prepare us for it. He was so nice, and I thanked him.

I left for a while to make calls, and found Burger King open. When I tried to crank the car, the battery was dead, so I called AAA. They were there in no time.

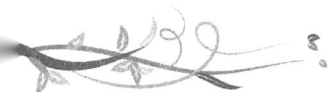

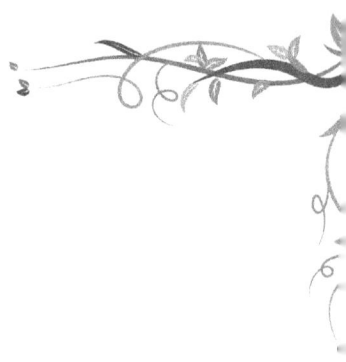

07/09/07 Monday

I stayed with Ken last night, and left about 5:00 am this morning. He had a fairly restful night. He got strangled a few times, but would go back to sleep. I came home, as I had several things to take care of. I called Ombudsman in reference to last Sunday's episode. I spoke with Sylvia, as Ashley the former Ombudsman referred me to her. Needless to say Sylvia was appalled, and said she would get right on it. She felt as I, that one week should be sufficient to have solved the issue.

Each time that I have called the nursing home, I am told that she's still reviewing, or either I have to leave a message. Hospice is waiting on the x-ray report, and blood work. Ken was so helpless today. He has Ativan ordered as needed, but it appears that no one will give this extra to him.

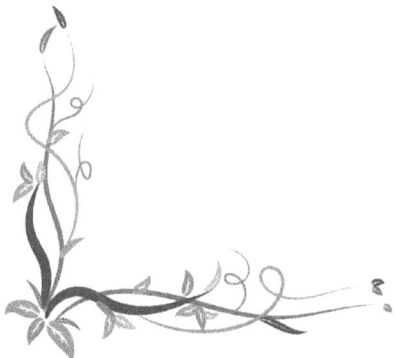

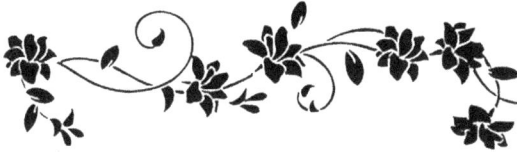

GOD'S ALMIGHTY PLAN

Have you ever watched a loved one dying in pain?
Did tears begin to flow as you tried to help in vain?
Did you stay near and hold their hands,
trying to understand God's Almighty plan?
Did you then remember His words,
"I'll never leave you nor forsake you,"
as you felt the presence of the Holy Spirit circumference the room?
Did you begin to see hands reaching toward the sky,
when a home sick look appeared in their eyes?
You now realize that it's not you,
but God who is holding their hands, as
He leads them into the Promised Land.

07/09/07

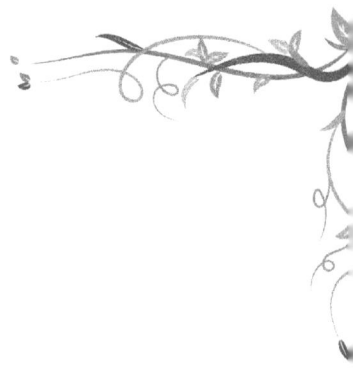

7/10/07 Tuesday

I am so sleepy. It's 12:00 a.m. I met with Hospice this morning at 11:30 a.m. I didn't sleep well last night. Both of my legs were cramping during the night, and I'd get up and rub them until the cramp would leave. I'd go back to bed, and then have to get back up.

I was so tired this morning that I was late leaving for the meeting. It went well. Both of the ladies were so nice. They reviewed what they had on file. The name of the funeral home had been changed from what I had given, and the person to be called had been changed. I knew who did it. The employee had called and apologized to me as he had been talking with a member of the family, rather than with me. I'm sure that was when the information was changed.

Ken will have a volunteer to sit with him. I'm not sure of the times, but I was told they are available. I will definitely feel better knowing that someone is with him, when I'm not. He has had another rough day. I have noticed that since we found him hanging out of the wheelchair, he has had little use of his right hand. I feel there has been nerve damage.

I noticed this afternoon that Ken would try to move it, and then he picked it up with his left hand. Something tells me that it is hurting him, and he's not able to tell me, but convincing staff of that is nigh to impossible. I mentioned this to one of the Hospice nurses, and she seemed to think it was alright.

I met the speech therapist this morning at the same time I met the Hospice ladies. She seems to know what she is talking about. She said that Ken chokes even on the honey-thickened liquids. If I understood her correctly, she recommended that he be taken off of any medicine that had to be given with a liquid. She said he is aspirating. The x-ray taken yesterday was negative for pneumonia. She said that could change at any time.

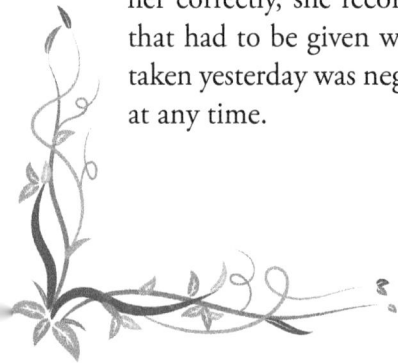

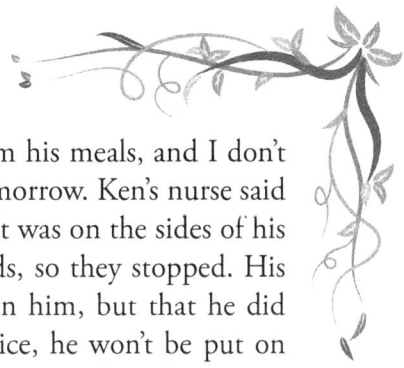

The nursing home is still trying to feed him his meals, and I don't understand it. I will talk with Lacy about it tomorrow. Ken's nurse said that at lunch Ken wasn't swallowing his food. It was on the sides of his mouth, and he also would choke on his liquids, so they stopped. His nurse said at supper that they got very little in him, but that he did alright with his medicine. According to Hospice, he won't be put on morphine until he declines more. I feel so helpless watching him try to eat and drink.

I went to work for about three hours this afternoon, and then went back to the nursing home. I wet one of the little sponges, and when I put it in Ken's mouth, he just sucked on it. I did this several times while I was there. When I began reading the Bible to him, he began making noises, and moving his legs and his left arm, and then tried to reach upward as he sat up in the bed. His eyes were looking up. As he fell back on the bed, I talked to him about Heaven and how beautiful it must be.

He sleeps most of the time, except when he becomes choked on his saliva. It's very frightening for him. I didn't get home until 10:00 p.m. It was hard to leave him, but I knew that I needed the rest to keep functioning. If I give out, it won't help Ken or me. He isn't moving nearly as much as he was. He just sort of lays there.

The Activities Director, brought a nature sound recording into Ken's room, and I pushed the night sounds. Ken moved his head some and I asked him if he thought he was at the tobacco barn curing tobacco. It also appeared that he recognized her voice. She has called him "Pretty Eyes" ever since he's been there. I walked with her to the hallway. She and I both cried. I played the sounds different times for him. I also played his CD music.

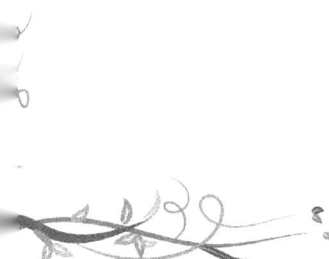

07/11/07 Wednesday

Lewana cut my hair this morning, and then followed me to see Ken. He was lying in bed looking so helpless.

The CNA he had this morning followed me into his room, and said that she normally works on another floor. She didn't know that she wasn't supposed to get Ken out of the bed, until after she had dressed him and gone to the dining room. She was told that he wasn't supposed to be dressed and not to get him out of bed. She said she took him back to bed, and put his gown on. **So much for communication!** Before I left tonight, someone had made a sign that was put over the bed that he is to be kept in bed, and in a gown.

The Hospice nurses aid came to see Ken, and asked me about his medicine and tube feeding. Of course, this has been discussed before, but there is always the chance the family member's feelings could change. The main nurse also came, and talked to him some. He smiled at her a little, and she said he knows what is happening. I told her the fact that he can't eat or drink is so hard, but at the same time watching him get choked and fighting for his breath is also hard. She said he doesn't appear to need to be put on the Morphine (Rexanal). He is getting so much weaker. He hasn't eaten more than 50% since the wheelchair incident. Most days, he eats very little, and gets choked. The nurse told me that he is aspirating, and she felt that all medication should be stopped. She was concerned about his seizure medication being stopped. She stated that she would call his doctor.

I spoke with the manager on 5th floor, and she said that he would be given Tylenol every 4 hours, and oxygen. When the CNA, took his temperature, it was 100.8. His nurse gave him a suppository Tylenol before I left. He said, "I'm not telling you what to do, but you need to go home and get some rest, because you may need it later." *I feel better about leaving Ken with the nurse and the CNA who is working.*

One of the CNA's came and had a book entitled "There is a Heaven." She sang When We All Get to Heaven, and then read from the book. I asked her to sing some more for us. She did, and we talked about when we accepted Christ as our Savior, and how the songs are different today than when we were young.

Ken seemed to enjoy her singing. She has sung for us many times. I would ask her to sing a particular song, and she knew them. I began to sing one of the songs, and she said, "that's not the way we sing it." I laughed, and told her that I was used to people kidding and laughing about my singing, but I just couldn't believe she had said that. We both had a good laugh, and I certainly enjoyed her visit.

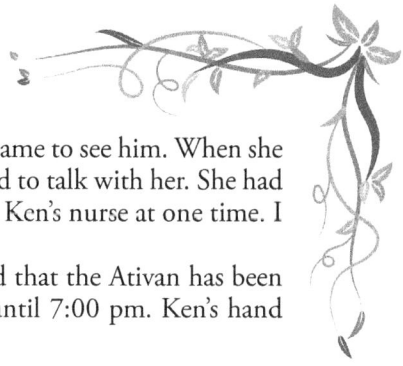

One of Ken's former nurses from another floor came to see him. When she called him by his name, he moved his head, and tried to talk with her. She had worked on this floor for several years, and had been Ken's nurse at one time. I thought it was so sweet of her to come see him.

I called the nursing home tonight, and was told that the Ativan has been ordered. I left about 3:00 pm, and went to work until 7:00 pm. Ken's hand still seems to be bothering him today.

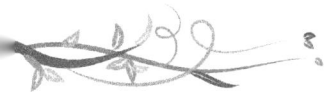

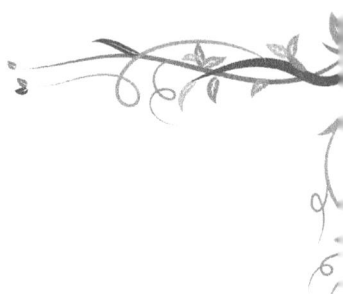

July 12, 2007 Thursday

When I got up this morning, I was so sleepy, even though I rested well. I just didn't get enough hours in. I had an appointment with my ophthalmologist for a follow-up visit from my glaucoma surgery. I came home, and put in some clothes to wash, cleaned out the car, and then took my shower. I had told Alecia, Ken's niece that I would meet her at 2:45 pm, and I didn't want to be late.

When we got to Ken's room, Susie, Alecia's mother was looking out the window. I quietly pulled the door to, and told Alecia for her to do what she wanted. She said, "I came to see Uncle Ken and that's what I'm going to do." When we walked in, and Susie saw us, it was like walking into a refrigerator. I spoke to her, and asked how she was doing, and she said, "Fine." She went to Ken's right side of the bed toward the floor, and she was between me and him. It appeared that she was in some way trying to keep me away from him. I asked her if he had been asleep, and she said. "I woke him up two or three times." I'm thinking, "Why do you think they gave him his medicine?"

The family has made it clear that they wanted no communication with me. I could have told her about the extra medication that helped him rest better. She also should have known by now that he needed to sleep; and not have to be told ! He is a sick man, and Shellie (associated with Hospice) told me that the morphine would help him breathe better. Shellie and I talked by cell on my way back from Mt. Airy. Susie was very cold toward me and Alecia, as if we weren't supposed to be there.

Ken was given his first dose of morphine at 1:30 pm. His nurse said it was so hard for him to do it, and his CNA was with him. He said they spent about twenty minutes with Ken before giving it to him. They both came back in before they left to go home, and spent some more time talking to him, and touching his face. They will be off until next Tuesday. His nurse gave me his cell number to call if anything happens before then.

My understanding was that the medicine would be administered

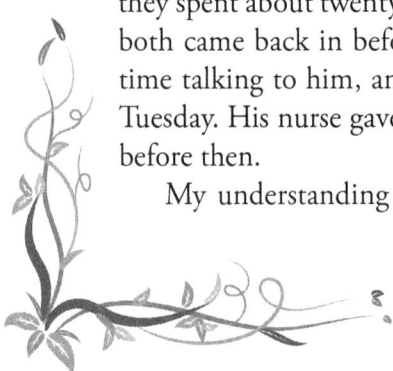

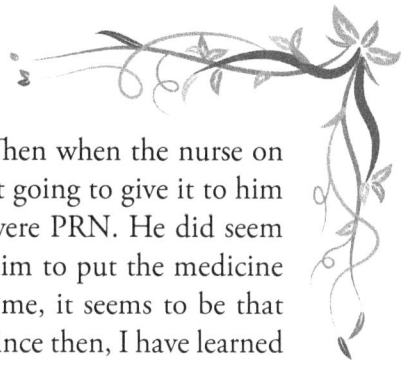

every 4 hours, and increased as he needed it. Then when the nurse on 3rd shift came in to see him, she said she wasn't going to give it to him until he got restless, because the instructions were PRN. He did seem to be resting well, and it may have disturbed him to put the medicine under his tongue. I'm no doctor, but at this time, it seems to be that giving this on a regular basis would be better. (Since then, I have learned that once morphine is activated, it should not be discontinued or doses skipped.) He has to be suctioned often, and his mouth cleaned out with the little sponges. He looked so much better today, than he did last night when I left.

Susie said that the nurse told her Monday that Ken only weighed one hundred twenty three pounds. She said they had done x-rays, and that he had a seizure while she was there. I asked her if she told the nurse, and she responded rather sharply that she did. I asked her for the nurse's name, and she said, "I don't know," but each time she used the word "she," not "him."

After she left, I spoke with the nurse, and told her what had been said. He does weigh a little over one hundred twenty three pounds according to his chart, but there was no mention of him having a seizure. I was given the name of the nurse who pulled a double shift Monday, so we have no way of knowing who told Susie. Alecia told her that Susie would have said she, even if it had been a he, because she knew she wasn't supposed to be told that information, because of the HIPPA law.

I told Shellie that I had been assured a long time ago that even though she was down as the emergency contact person, she was only to be called after they tried my work number, my home number, and my cell number, but evidently it wasn't done. I had her name taken off today. We had been there about thirty minutes when Susie decided she was leaving. Alecia and I stayed a while longer, and left. She and I stood outside the building and talked a long time. It was good for both of us. It's 3:00 a.m., and I need to get to bed.

I stayed with Ken until 12:00 am. When I left, he was holding Tigger in his hand. Tigger is a small stuffed animal. Some of the nurses and CNA's are good to open his hands, and put his fingers around Tigger, but some of them don't. It seems to comfort him. Anne gave this to him.

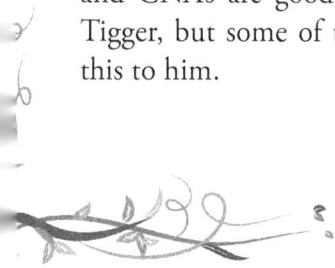

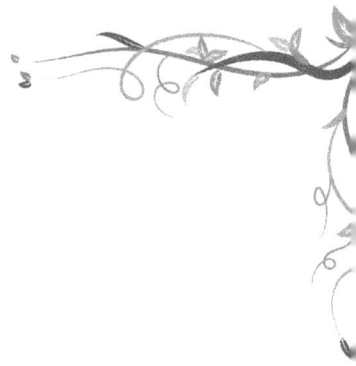

07/13/07 Friday

This has been a hard, tiresome week. When the alarm went off this morning, I thought it can't be time already. I ate breakfast, showered, and went to physical therapy. When I left there, I went to see Ken before going to work. I got there around 11:30 am. Ken was full of mucous.

I went down the hall, and asked his nurse, "How long has it been since you suctioned him out?" He said. "8:30 this morning." I responded with, "And it's 11:30 am now? You need to suction him, and the instrument that is to be put in the mouth is on the floor." He had to go to 4th floor to get another one. He got two, so he'd have an extra if needed.

I went downstairs and asked for the director of nursing. She was off today; so were the other two with whom I could speak with. I wound up talking to someone else whom I'd never met before. She tried to intimidate me. She said, "There may have been a good reason that the nurse hadn't suctioned him. Maybe he had to go to another floor to get the tube."

I questioned her as to why there wouldn't be any available for 5th floor, since they know there is a big possibility they would be needed. She asked me "Haven't you ever run out of toilet paper?" I just looked at her. She said, "If A didn't tell B that something needed to be ordered, then B wouldn't know they were out."

It seems to me that they would have someone to do a regular check to make sure that everything was stocked. Just like everything else, lack of communication. She asked me how often I thought Ken needed to be suctioned. I told her at least every hour to an hour 1/2. She said that is a reasonable request. She will follow up on this. At the same time, I got the impression that she wasn't overly concerned.

I called Ombudsman. She said tomorrow would be a good day to go to the Nursing Home. I have two appointments next week, and also two doctor appointments. It will be a busy week.

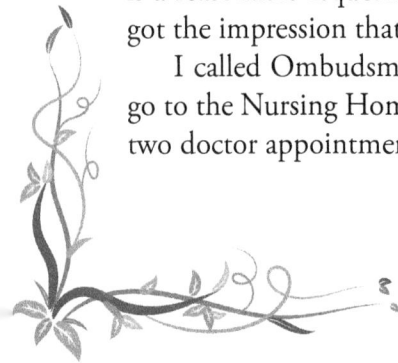

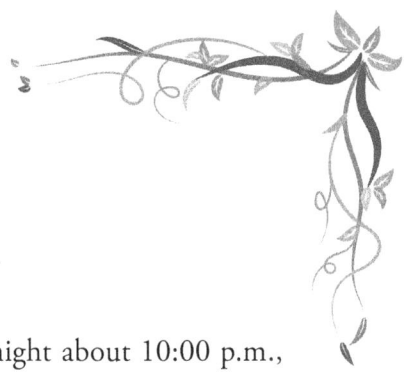

07/14/07 Saturday

I have had a busy day. I went to bed last night about 10:00 p.m., and I didn't wake up until 10:00 a.m. Lewana called to check on Ken. After that, I ate breakfast. I vacuumed, dusted, mopped, put in clothes to wash, and put two NY steaks on to cook. I had them in the freezer, and I was so glad, because I'm craving beef. I ate half of one and it was so good. I also ate a tomato sandwich that was good. After I was through with house cleaning, I took a shower, and washed my hair.

I left much later than I had planned to go see Ken. I went by the post office, and had put the trash in the car trunk. I forgot the dump closes at 4:00 on Saturday. I called my friend Donna, and she was on her way back from Charlotte. She had carried part of the church youth group to the airport. She said they were so excited. I told her about the trash in the trunk, and she said to leave it in front of the garage, and she'd put it with theirs to be picked up. Friends such as this are hard to find.

When I saw Ken, he was lying sort of comatose. There was no indication that he was aware of what his sister has said. I just sat in a chair beside the bed, and held his hand. Then he became fidgety, and began moving his legs. When his nurse took his temperature, he didn't have a fever. Later she listened to his lungs, and she could hear a little congestion. He looks worn out.

His sister, and her friend came to see him. His sister asked me, or rather stated in question form that he would be left at the nursing home, and not transferred to the Hospice House. I asked her who told her that. She said the nurse at hospice. (The nurse should have known not to share that information with anyone due to the HIPPA law.) I told her that originally, I had planned to move him there, after he no longer is aware of where he is. She came back loudly with, "I don't want him riding in one of them ambulances being bounced all over the place." I just looked at her, and said "I rode in the ambulance when Daddy was moved from the hospital to the Hospice House. The driver was very cautious, and it was a very smooth ride. I guessed it depended on the driver. Ken may not live long enough to move him."

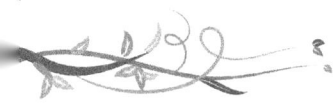

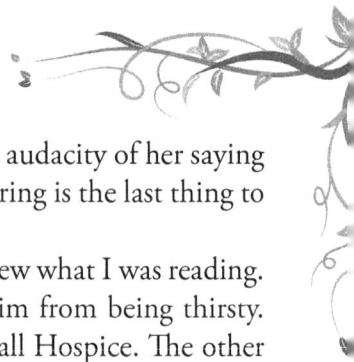

I was furious with her. I could not believe the audacity of her saying all of that in his presence, as if he wasn't there hearing is the last thing to leave before their last breathe.

I read some to him, but I couldn't tell if he knew what I was reading. I asked his nurse if IV fluids would help keep him from being thirsty. She said it would, and asked if I wanted her to call Hospice. The other nurse made the call, and they returned her call right away. The doctor ordered the IV, and the nurse brought the necessary equipment to his room that would be needed. The first vein blew, but the 2nd one was good.

Ken was finally given his morphine about 10:30. He lay with his eyes open for a long time, and finally went to sleep about 12:00. The CNA for 3rd shift came in to see him, and she was very nice. She said, "I've had Ken on other nights, and would check to see if he was wet, and he wouldn't be." The next time I checked him, he would be soaked. He is urinating very little because of his intake."

(I don't know enough about how much the IV's will affect the kidneys.) I left about 12:00 a.m. His nurse came in not long before that, and said he didn't have a fever, and his vitals were good, but that he sounded a little congested. This means that he is getting pneumonia. The 3rd shift nurse said she will call me if there is any change.

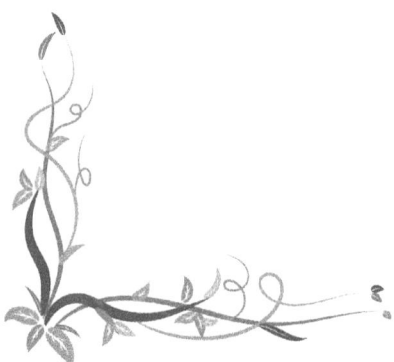

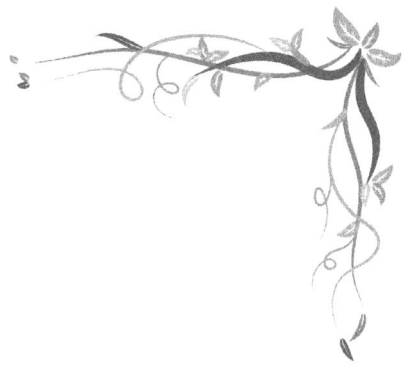

07/15/07 Sunday

I didn't sleep last night. I got up this morning about 10:00. I kept lying in the bed hoping I would go to sleep for a little while. Anne called me and said she would be here after church. I ate a little something to keep me from getting hungry. I called Susie to update her on Ken. Then, I called Mary, another friend who is taking chemo treatments. When Anne came in, she had a broccoli casserole, cream potatoes, cantaloupe, and baked apples. I had the steak and cornbread. We pooled our food together, and everything was so good. When we finished, we talked for a while, and then cleaned up the table, and loaded the dishwasher.

When she left, I went to see Ken. There is a drastic change from yesterday. His breathing is so much more difficult for him. His oxygen had already been increased, and he had a temperature this morning of 101. They gave him Tylenol suppositories, and when I left, it had come down to 99.7. That is still not good. His nurse gave him his morphine. She had given some to him at 6:00 a.m., but thought he needed it again. He just lies there with his eyes open. Once in a while, he'll move them, but if I move my hand back and forth in front of his eyes, he doesn't follow it.

When the CNA's changed his position, it pulled out his IV. His nurse called another nurse. She kept sticking him to find a good vein. I asked her to note that if it was pulled out again, to not reinsert it, because I didn't want him stuck so many times. I know how that hurts. Even though he has been getting the fluids, he is still dehydrated. She said this is normal for an end of life cycle. Later, I asked for Ken's chart. I thought it rather odd that there was nothing documented from 07/01/07 until 07/09/07.

When I left tonight, Ken had his eyes wide open, but I couldn't get him to look at me. I had read to him earlier, but he didn't show that he heard me.

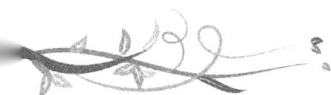

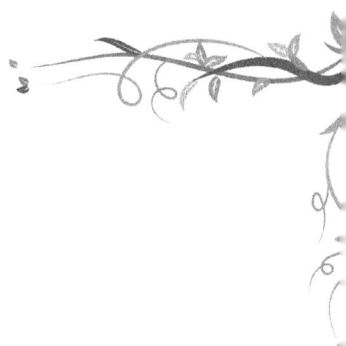

07/16/07 Monday

I didn't sleep again last night even though I went to bed. I tossed and turned all night, and then about 7:00 a.m. I went to sleep. I slept about two hours. I felt as if I wasn't going to make it when I got up. I thought that after my shower, I'd be wide awake. When anyone would ask me today about how I felt, I'd tell them that I was sleepwalking.

I went in to work about 1:30 p.m. and worked until 5:30 p.m. I went by the nursing home this morning, and stayed with Ken a while. I could tell that he is weaker today than yesterday. He is still getting his IV's. He just lets that arm lie straight beside him, and doesn't move it.

I think I'll ask his doctor if he will have it x-rayed.

They have given Ken morphine every 4 hours today. The nurse he has tonight doesn't give it to him like some of the other nurses do. She may not give it to him for 8 hours stating that he doesn't need it. I'm uneasy about him when she has him. He is having such difficulty breathing. The morphine should help him relax and breathe easier. If he is given too much, it won't be good, and won't help him later. I'm not sure when they think they will increase it. He is still lying real still with his eyes half open. He coughed a little one time, and rose up some, and then just lay back. I told the nurse, and she suctioned him out later, and he went to sleep.

Anne had called me earlier in the day, and told me to come by and eat supper. I left about 8:30 p.m., and she had ham biscuits and sweet potato pie that Jeanette had made. All tasted good. I am so sleepy, and I hope I can sleep when I go to bed.

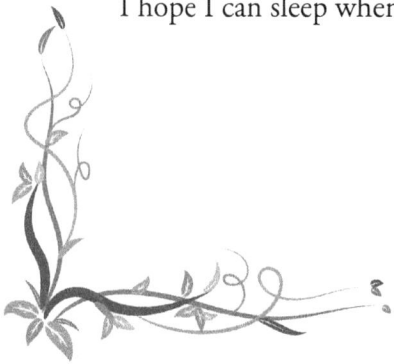

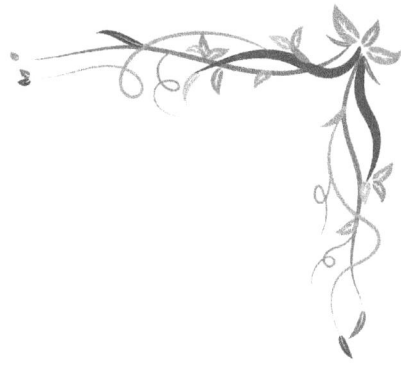

07/17/07 Tuesday

I couldn't sleep last night, and about 1:30 a.m., I got up and went back to the nursing home. I sat beside Ken's bed, and held his hand. It was so hard to listen to him trying to breathe. I would use the little sponges to moisten his mouth, and kept lip moisturizer on his lips.

His nurse was surprised that Ken was still alive, and that was because of the IV fluids. I asked that they be removed if OK with the doctor. I didn't want him to be kept alive in the shape he was in, just because of me. They were removed. He just seems to me to be getting weaker, even when the IV fluids were being given.

The Hospice nurse also said that the fluids could build up in his body, because his kidneys weren't able to dispose of as much liquid as his intake, and that would be worse than letting nature take its course. If this had been explained to me, I wouldn't have asked for the IV's..

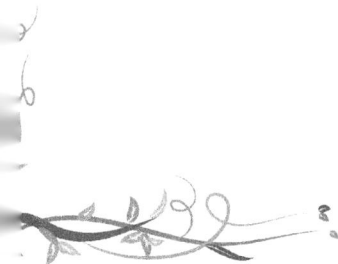

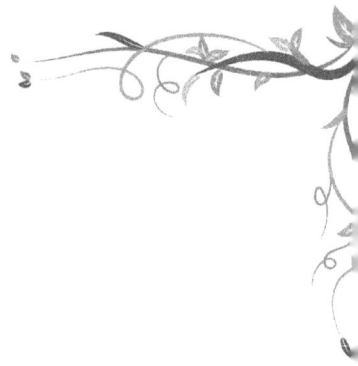

07/18/07 Wednesday

I stayed with Ken, as he is getting much worse, and I don't want to leave him. I feel at times he senses that I'm with him. His temperature has been 105 degrees. I have kept cold cloths on his forehead, and bathed his face, neck and chest to give him some relief. He has lost the ability to hold his head straight.

Each time he has been repositioned, they are placing extra padding to make him more comfortable, and keeping the head of the bed raised up. His CNA came in and put sheets on the extra bed, and told me that I needed to rest, and I could stay with him as long as I wanted to.

Alecia came when she got off of work. She took me out to eat, and it was so good. I didn't realize that I was that hungry. She stayed with me until about 11:00 p.m. I told Alecia to go on home to her family, and that I'd be fine. She did have me to rest a while earlier. I dozed for about thirty minutes which seemed to really help me. This was so considerate of her and so much appreciated.

After Alecia left, I tried to rest, but I couldn't. I kept getting up to check on Ken. I finally got up and stayed up. He never did close his eyes as if he was resting, even though he was being given his morphine every four hours. His breathing never seemed to improve. I finally decided to leave about 5:00 a.m.

The Ombudsman came to see Ken for the first time, and watched him for a long time. I then got the chart for her, and she was concerned also that there was no documentation from 07/01/07 through 07/08/07. She said if this were to be subpoenaed to court that the nursing home would be in big trouble.

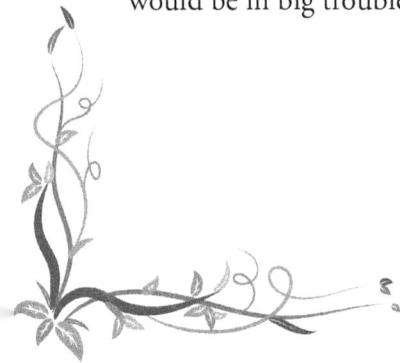

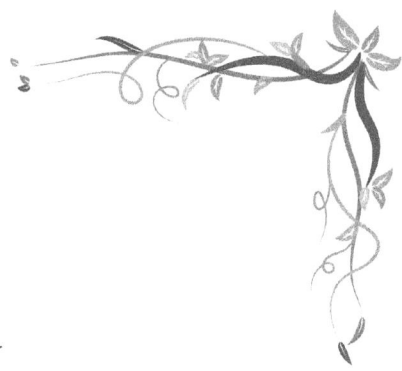

07/19/07 Thursday

I ate some breakfast this morning, and went to bed hoping to rest a little, even if I didn't sleep. I slept about 2 hours, and then got three different phone calls. I had already decided that I'd get up and go back to Ken, when Hospice called. I hurried and took my shower, then left.

Four Hospice nurses were standing on the left side of his bed watching him. Two of his nurses, along with his CNA, were standing on his right. They got some ice bags, wrapped in a towel, and put under his arms. His temperature was 105 degrees. His respiration was 44 and should have been 20. He was really suffering. They finally got permission to give the morphine every hour, but he passed away. He took one breath with almost a groan and then died. (I'm not sure what time he died. I think about 12:00 pm and he was just 62 years old.)

I asked Crystal with Hospice to call Susie, and Lewana, who told her she would call Alecia. I was so thankful for Chaplain Walker, and all of the Hospice family who were so supportive throughout the whole ordeal. I had written a poem about Ken entitled Until Then. I shared it with them, and they seemed to understand.

I told Mr. Walker that when Ken's family came in, that I would give them some private time. I went downstairs to get a drink with Alecia, who had arrived during this time. We waited for Lewana. When she came in, we went back to his room. Teddy and Sarah came in first, then Susie and Delight. Teddy and Sarah left before we went back upstairs.

The funeral home hearse was to be there at 2:00 p.m. I didn't leave until after the body was moved. Alecia had to go back to work, and Lewana followed me home. She went with me to the funeral home to finalize everything. Barry (funeral home attendant) wanted me to go to the cemetery to make sure they had the right plot. We did that, and then Lewana and I drove to the house where Ken and I had lived, for approximately eight years. She remembered the house from when she was a child, but didn't know where it was.

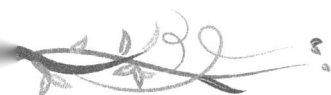

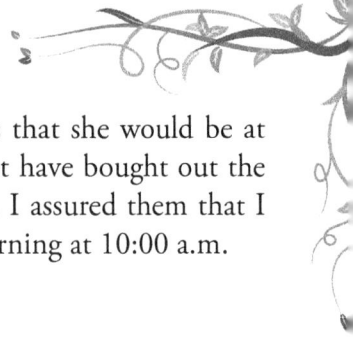

Laura called on our way home, and told us that she would be at my house by the time we were. I think she must have bought out the grocery store. She and Lewana stayed until late. I assured them that I would be alright. Lewana will be back in the morning at 10:00 a.m.

ROMANS 8: 38,39

FOR I AM PERSUADED, THAT NEITHER DEATH, NOR LIFE NOR ANGELS, NOR PRINCIPALITIES, NOR POWER, NOR THINGS PRESENT, NOR THINGS TO COME, NOR HEIGHT, NOR DEPTH, NOR ANY OTHER CREATURE, SHALL BE ABLE TO SEPARATE US FROM THE LOVE OF GOD, WHICH IS IN CHRIST JESUS, OUR LORD.

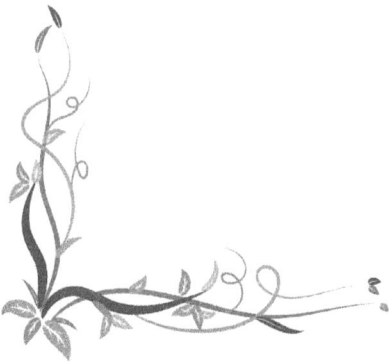

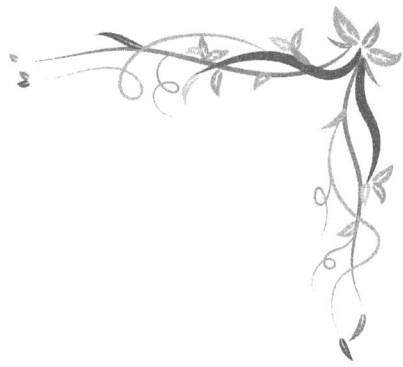

07/20/07 Friday

I slept good last night. I guess I was so exhausted. Lewana and I went to the funeral home. She wanted to make sure Ken's hair and everything was alright, before his family arrived for the viewing. A dear cousin, Jewell, was at the house early this morning. She followed me and Lewana to the funeral home. I was pleased with how they had prepared Ken's body.

When his family came, Alexandria told me she was pleased with the choices that I had made. She said the spray on the casket was the prettiest she had ever seen. Nothing was said to me about anything being wrong with the obituary. I asked the family to go back by the house for a while, but they wanted to go home. They said they would meet me at the funeral home for visitation tonight.

Alecia arrived at the house about 4:00 p.m. Somewhere along the way, Barry called and said that a female had called the newspaper five times to get them to change information in the obituary. The paper has a policy that nothing will be printed or changed, unless the information comes on funeral home letterhead fax. Barry wondered if I knew who may have made the call. I didn't know who did, but knew it wasn't me.

He decided to wait until visitation. He was with me in the visitation parlor. As he stepped out the door (as he later told) he was confronted by Susie that the full name of their mother needed to be changed, the middle name of their father needed to be changed, one of the brothers' middle name needed to be included, etc. I had already been asked if the husband's names were included with the sister's name in parenthesis.

He didn't know that they had already stopped at his office, and asked the secretary to change all of this on the funeral home information. He told her he would be glad to fax the newspaper the new information, but it would cost $150.00, and that I had already paid for everything. If they wanted it changed, he would need to know the name and address

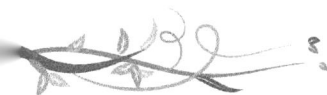

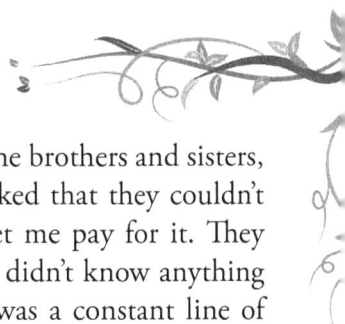

of the person to be billed. She went back to ask the brothers and sisters, and then told him to just leave it. He was shocked that they couldn't come up with the money, and was willing to let me pay for it. They never mentioned this to me, and thought that I didn't know anything about it. I never mentioned it to them. There was a constant line of people who came to pay their respect.

Barry came with some cold water for me. I didn't realize that my mouth was so dry. I really appreciated the number of people who shared remembrances with me, and many whom I hadn't seen in a long time. I was so thankful that my feet didn't prevent me from being there. It was unnerving to see Ken in the casket.

Alecia and Lewana insisted they were taking me to the funeral home. It was comforting to have them with me. I was so tired when I got home, but I couldn't seem to unwind enough to go to sleep. On the way back home, Alecia and Lewana, both asked who was the beautiful black haired girl who was sitting in the lobby. They said she was sobbing her heart out. I told them that no one who looked like that came through the line. No one who resembled the description.

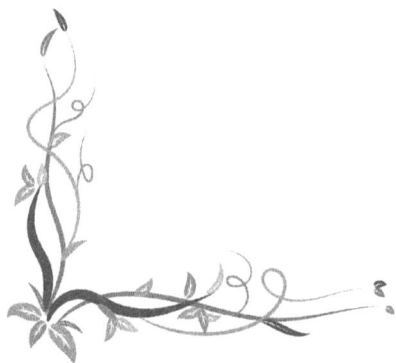

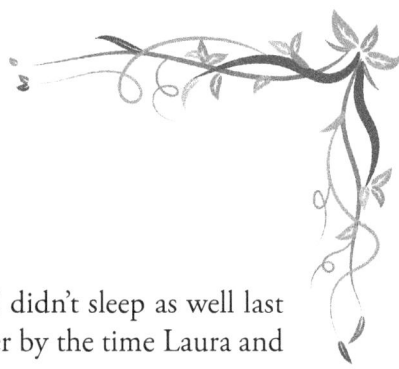

07/21/07

Saturday, I was up by 9:00 a.m. although I didn't sleep as well last night as I had hoped. I wanted to get my shower by the time Laura and Lewana came. They took such good care of me.

I had mentioned that I wanted to go back to the funeral home one more time. Laura said she would take me, and then deliver some of the food to the church that Lewana had brought. She came back by to get me. By the time we returned, Lewana had put everything in the freezer. By now, it was time for us to dress for the funeral.

Barry said he would pick us up at 1:30. I was very nervous. When we arrived at the church, Ken's family was waiting for us. Barry lined us up to walk into the church. Laura was on one side of me, and Lewana was on the other. It was so hard to walk down the aisle. It was such a different feeling from when I walked down the aisle almost 41 years ago to be married.

Gerald and his sister, Linda, had fixed a CD of Ken being accompanied by Karen Byrd singing and me playing the piano. I'm not sure which songs he chose, but I heard the last part of "I've Come Too Far to Look Back," just before we walked in. It was almost my undoing.

Gerald and Wayne did such a wonderful job with their comments, and also asking if there was anyone who hadn't made a decision to follow Jesus needed to do so. I've known both of them since they were little fellows. It makes me feel old, but very proud of them. Angel and Jeff sang the two songs previously requested by Ken to be sung at his funeral. Their voices harmonized beautifully. When the service was over, the Ladies of the church fed us in the Fellowship Hall. It was well appreciated.

When we were finished with our meal, Barry drove us to the cemetery to view the grave. It still doesn't seem real. When we were ready to leave, Barry drove me, Laura, and Lewana back to my house. They left then to go to their homes. I asked Ken's family if they wanted to come back by the house, but they said no.

Later in the day, Anne came and we had supper together. It was nice to be able to relax and try to unwind. Evenings are the hardest, for this was when I went to see Ken at the nursing home.

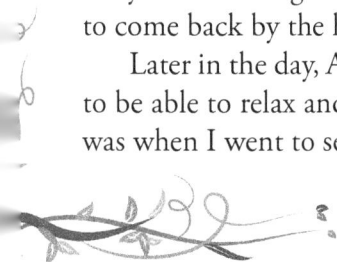

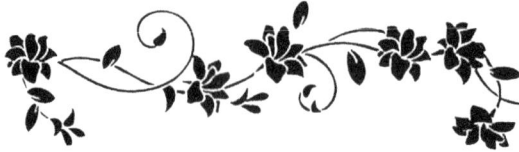

WHERE DO I GO?

Where do I go from here?
My life is in such disarray.
and I have to face it
come what may.
Sometimes it feels as if
I'm in the depth of the sea
with the water covering me.
I begin fighting to get to the top;
not sure if I want to as
I begin to rise to the surface.
A small voice whispers,
You are here for a purpose

11/18/04

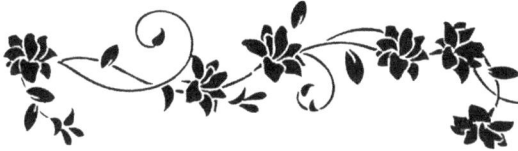

NO ONE

I feel so sad and alone,
needing someone to call my own.
I need to be loved, touched, and held.
No one to share thoughts with,
no one to tell.
My life was once an open book.
Now, it's so empty,
I'm afraid to look.

11/18/04

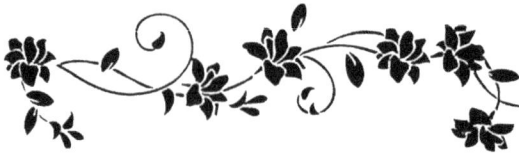

BEING PATIENT

Sometimes we have to wait our turn.
This is a lesson that's so hard to learn.
As children we would push and shove,
forgetting the lessons taught about love.
We become impatient waiting for answers.
God's ways are not our ways,
and His time is not our time.
Sometimes we lay awake all night.
Then, in His own time,
He makes everything alright.

03/10/05

We think we can help God by
Giving Him a shove.

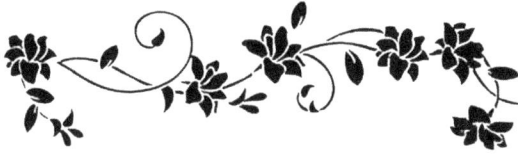

THE COLOR OF GRAY

You stand there in front of me
but you're not there
The color of gray are your eyes
as you stand with such a confused look
on your face with no one near
to help you escape
In this photograph of you in my mind
you are wearing your blue and gray
jacket that matches your eyes
and is faded with age
Your eyes that were once blue
now are gray
There is a jagged hole torn in the elbow
of the jacket that has molded to
fit the shape of your body and
has grown old with you
Each time I come in contact with the
soft warm comfortable cloth
it has an aroma of tobacco smoke
As your life comes to an end
the confused look will go away
Your eyes will again turn peaceful blue
and will no longer be the color of gray

2000

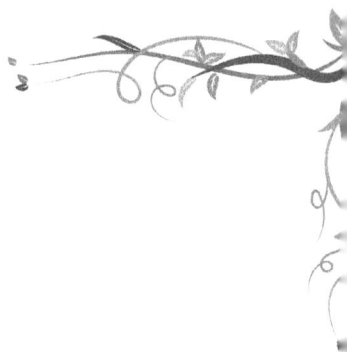

As I sit quietly reflecting on the events prior to Ken's death, I'm reminded of my Heavenly Father's promise, "I'll never leave you nor forsake you."

I requested early disability retirement to become effective June 30, 2008, due to overall health problems. Prior to that on May 16, 2008, I fell at work, and broke my right wrist, and had to have surgery, and physical therapy. On July 05, 2008, I twisted my left leg, and broke the tibia bone on my right leg. I was in a wheelchair for six weeks. Over time, these healed, but I was still dealing with a torn rotator cuff from the May 16, 2008, fall. I eventually had surgery which didn't hold. There's been quite a bit of adjusting. I keep telling myself, that this too, shall pass.

It took several months for me to heal physically and mentally after Ken's death.

I have spent several hours assembling all of the documentation that I had kept during Ken's illness which covered 15 years. The Lord has opened many doors for me, and allowed me to share encouragement with so many people who were hurting.

I am now playing the organ in church, and I also play piano at home. This has been such good therapy for me, as I lose track of time and concerns. I can't play for hours as I once did (because of my wrist and shoulder), but I can still play.

I enjoy opportunities that I have to listen to my brother play guitar. I also enjoy visiting with my nieces and nephews, and friends.

I have been so blessed.

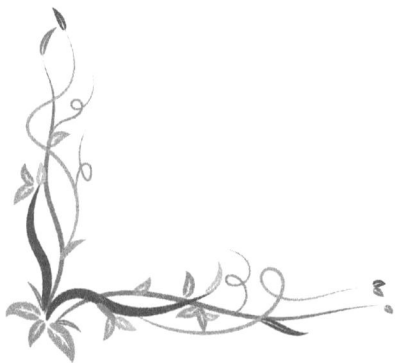

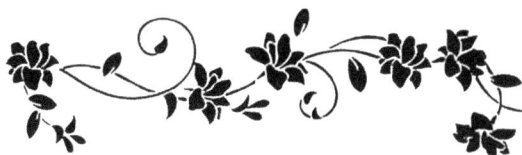

FINAL CHAPTER OF CLOSURE
07/20/24

This is the final chapter of just a portion, of what our marriage consisted of for almost 41 years. There were many happy times, sad, gut wrenching, and emotional moments. We shared these together, and separately. For me, so many questions with no answers; Ken, also had questions with no answers. I have dealt with some of them already, but not all.

The person whom I thought I was marrying; was not the same person I knew, and who I fell in love with. I have heard of people who have developed different personalities. This happens in order to function with situations they can't adhere to.

As time rolled by, I would catch a glimpse of the one I was familiar with. As years came, and went, there were pronounced differences. There were more things happening, and therefore; more doctors, and more tests in order to confirm the diagnoses.

Before and after Ken was diagnosed, different issues were brought into the time-frame... It was factual that he had been unfaithful in our marriage. I felt that Ken and the Lord had resolved this issue, and was at peace.

Ken had childhood issues with sexual and physical abuse that was unknown to the doctors, when he was originally diagnosed with Alzheimer's. The doctor stated he never matured past his teen years. I have to keep reminding myself that mentally, he never matured beyond teenage years. I was more enlightened, as I began to connect dots.

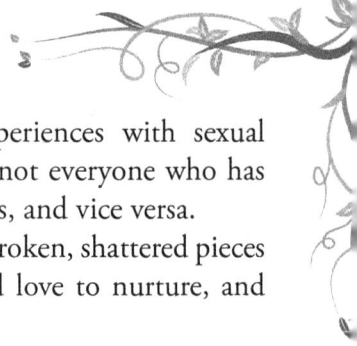

Although I have discussed Ken's past experiences with sexual abuse and Alzheimer's, it is important to note, not everyone who has experienced sexual abuse will develop Alzheimer's, and vice versa.

God with His infinite wisdom, mended the broken, shattered pieces back together. He gave me the compassion and love to nurture, and meet Ken's… needs.

After much struggle with myself, and God, I know there is a reason that this information is to be included. I don't have to know the reason. May the Lord use what is within these pages to bless.

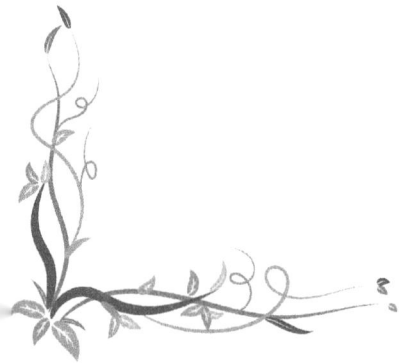

Milton Keynes UK
Ingram Content Group UK Ltd.
UKHW031000231024
450026UK00011B/697